Hands-On Thread Embedding Therapy

A Manual for Chronic Pain Treatment
Through Structural Stabilization

K-Medicine Academy

About the Authors

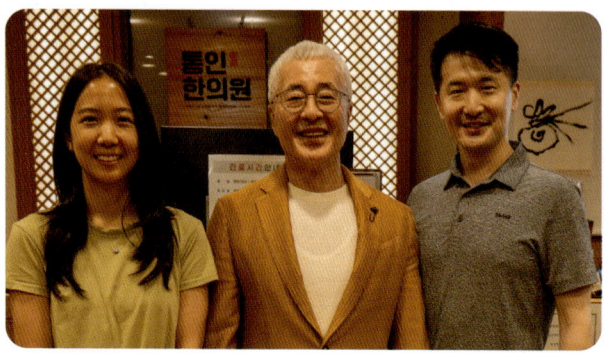

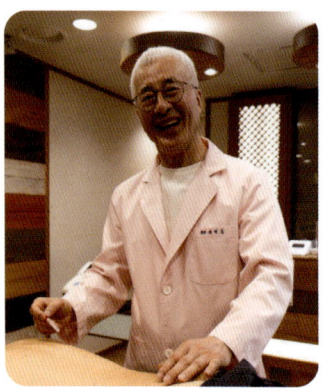

Byung-il Choi

Korean Medicine Doctor

Graduated from the College of Korean Medicine and completed graduate coursework at Kyung Hee University.

Former Medical Director at Donggang Korean Medicine Hospital (Specialized in integrative care between Western and Korean medicine)

Former Member of the Society of Pathologists

Current Director of Choi Byung-Il 3S Korean Medicine Clinic

Current Member of the Pathology Society of Korean Medicine

Founder and President of the Korean Association of Thread Embedding Acupuncture for Pain

* Approved for Excellent Clinical Technique by the Korea Institute of Oriental Medicine (KIOM) for "Thread Embedding Acupuncture for Low Back Pain and Radiating Leg Pain"
* Principal Investigator of the pilot study: "Efficacy and Safety of Thread Embedding Acupuncture on Chronic Low Back Pain" – foundational technology for clinical application
* Holder of a domestic patent and international applications (including China) for a Thread Embedding Acupuncture insertion device; PCT (Patent Cooperation Treaty) application submitted.

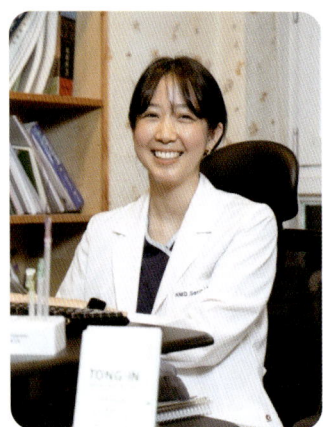

Serin Lee (@roveshin)

Korean Medicine Doctor

Chair, 2024 School Doctor Program Committee, Jongno District, Seoul

Chair, 2023 Senior Health Promotion Program Committee, Jongno District, Seoul

Vice Chair, Public Relations Committee for Korean Medicine Clinic at the 2023 Saemangeum World Scout Jamboree

Publications:

「Safe and Effective Use of Long Needles」
「Hands-On Long Needle Technique: Korean Acupuncture」
「Hands-On Korean Cosmetic Acupuncture」
「Before You Turn Eleven: What You Need to Know About Your Body」
「Before You Turn Fourteen: Understanding Body and Mind」
「Guidebook for Attracting Southeast Asian Medical Tourists to Korean Medicine Clinics」

About the Authors

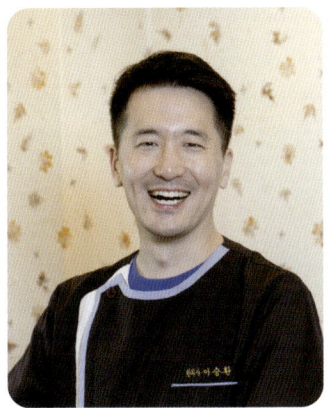

Seung Hwan Lee (@wooricare)
Korean Medicine Doctor
Ph.D. in Preventive Korean Medicine, Kyung Hee University
M.S. in Women's Korean Medicine, Dongguk University
Licensed Acupuncturist, State of New York, USA

Chief Director, Tong-in Korean Medicine Clinic
President, Jongno District Association of Korean Medicine
Chair, School Doctor Program Committee, Seoul Association of Korean Medicine
Vice Chair, Pediatric and Adolescent Committee, Association of Korean Medicine (AKOM)

Publications:
「Safe and Effective Use of Long Needles」
「Hands-On Long Needle Technique: Korean Acupuncture」
「Hands-On Korean Cosmetic Acupuncture」
「Practical Guide to Classical Prescriptions in Korean Medicine」
「English Consultation Guide for Korean Medicine Doctors and Students」
「K-Medicine for My Family」
「Guidebook for Attracting Southeast Asian Medical Tourists to Korean Medicine Clinics」
「Before You Turn Eleven: What You Need to Know About Your Body」
「Before You Turn Fourteen: Understanding Body and Mind」
「Prevention Made Easy: A Korean Medicine Approach」
「Who? Korean History Series: Heo Jun」
「It's Just Stress」

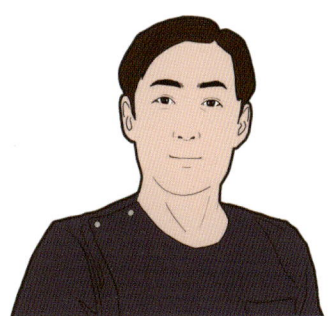

Kyungmin Chu (@callidesign04)
Korean Medicine Doctor & Medical Illustrator
Founder & Creative Director of calliDesign
Bridging Korean Medicine and Visual Design through medical illustration and creative communication.

Publications:
「K-Medicine for My Family」

Recommendation

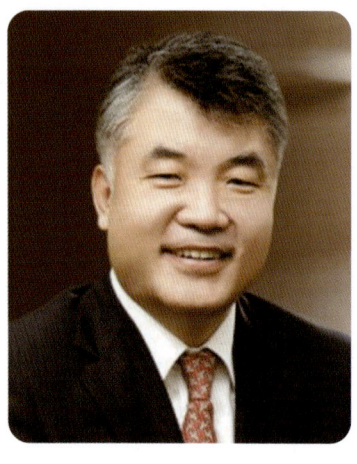

It is with great pleasure that I join you in celebrating the publication of "Hands-On Thread Embedding Therapy: A Manual for Chronic Pain Treatment Through Structural Stabilization"

Thread Embedding Acupuncture is a modern advancement in Korean medicine, developed to enhance the therapeutic effects of traditional acupuncture. This book is expected to serve as an invaluable guide for healthcare professionals seeking to learn and apply this technique.

Grounded in extensive clinical experience in the field of pain management, the manual offers a structured presentation of practical techniques and real-world clinical applications, making it both accessible and highly applicable for practitioners.

Authored by Dr. Byung-il Choi—one of the foremost experts in Thread Embedding Acupuncture both in Korea and internationally—this book is poised to open new horizons in pain treatment through the use of this innovative method.

I look forward to the continued advancement and wider clinical adoption of Thread Embedding Acupuncture and hope that many readers will find this book a valuable tool for delivering effective pain relief.

With sincere encouragement and warm congratulations on this achievement.

Summer 2025
In Boston

Seunghoon Choi, KMD
Honorary President, International Society of Oriental Medicine (ISOM)
Director, Massachusetts Integrative Medicine Center

Endorsement

Chronic musculoskeletal instability not only causes pain—it disrupts daily function and creates a vicious cycle that degrades quality of life.

Dr. Choi Byung-Il recognized earlier than most that true healing requires more than simply blocking pain signals; it demands a structural and integrative approach. His years of heartfelt dedication to each and every patient have left a deep impression on us all.

From the early days when even the term "thread embedding" was unfamiliar, he has refined this therapy through visionary insight and relentless clinical inquiry. Now, the wisdom and clinical experience he has accumulated over decades have been distilled into this remarkable book.

'Hands-On Thread Embedding Therapy: A Manual for Chronic Pain Treatment Through Structural Stabilization' is more than a technical guide—it is a profound testament to how a physician should approach their patients, both in practice and in spirit.

I sincerely hope this invaluable book serves as a guiding light for many healthcare professionals and patients alike.

Hyunjung Kwon, MD
Professor, Department of Anesthesiology and Pain Medicine
Seoul Asan Medical Center

Tribute

Heartfelt congratulations on the publication of Dr. Choi Byung-Il's book—an extraordinary culmination of his lifelong passion and profound insight, marking a new chapter in the treatment of musculoskeletal pain.

As a son who had grown up and, over time, perhaps grown distant, your unwavering dedication to thread embedding therapy became an invaluable "moment of reunion." The days we spent discussing and studying together—me, a fledgling medical student—were more than academic exchanges. They remain among the warmest memories of my life, moments when a father and son truly met and came to understand one another.

While many understood thread embedding therapy as merely a traditional technique involving the insertion of threads into acupuncture points, you had already envisioned something far beyond. Grounded in a deep anatomical understanding of the musculoskeletal system, you sought to restore structural balance and functional stability. This was not just an evolution of existing practice—it was a bold redefinition of therapeutic principles.

As your son, and as a fellow physician following in your footsteps, I am deeply proud of this book, which encapsulates your remarkable journey. I hope it offers inspiration to many healthcare professionals and relief to countless patients.

With deepest respect and love,
Your son, June Ho Choi
Professor of Neurosurgery, Asan Medical Center, Seoul

Your daughter-in-law, Hyunjung Kwon
Professor of Anesthesiology and Pain Medicine, Asan Medical Center, Seoul

Your daughter, Chanhyo Choi
Resident, Department of Anesthesiology and Pain Medicine, Kyungpook National University Hospital

Preface

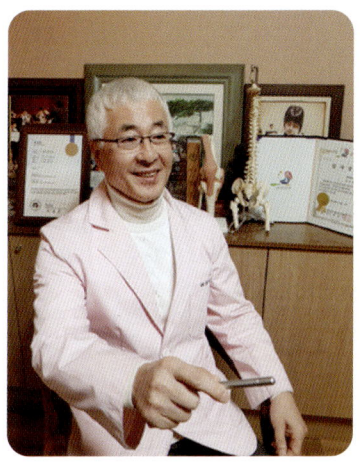

It has already been over a decade since I began teaching structural Thread Embedding Acupuncture for pain management.

While preparing a proper clinical manual, I had the great fortune of meeting Dr. Seung Hwan Lee and Dr. Serin Lee.

Through our collaboration, we were able to publish the first edition of this clinical manual on Thread Embedding Acupuncture — and I am deeply grateful and delighted by the outcome.

I promise to continue sharing more clinical know-how through future publications, and I reaffirm my commitment to the advancement of clinical techniques in Thread Embedding Acupuncture, as well as efforts toward the establishment of an official academic society, an international conference, and eventual inclusion in national health insurance coverage.

Thank you.

Sep. 2025.

Lead Author
Byung-il Choi, KMD
President, Korean Association of Thread Embedding Acupuncture for Pain

Table of Contents

About the Authors   ⋯   1 p
Recommendation   ⋯   3 p
Endorsement   ⋯   4 p
Tribute   ⋯   5 p
Preface   ⋯   6 p

Ⅰ. Thread Embedding Acupuncture
   1. Overview and History of Thread Embedding Acupuncture   ⋯   9 p
   2. Theoretical Foundations of Thread Embedding Acupuncture
      1) Relationship Between Meridian Theory and Thread Embedding   ⋯   9 p
      2) Anatomical Basis for Thread Embedding Acupuncture   ⋯   10 p
      3) Application of Thread Embedding Acupuncture to Trigger Points   ⋯   10 p
   3. Mechanisms of Action   ⋯   10 p
   4. Clinical Efficacy of Thread Embedding Acupuncture
      1) Enhanced Function of Muscle Spindles & Golgi Tendon Organs   ⋯   11 p
      2) Fusimotor Reflex   ⋯   11 p
      3) Collagen Regeneration   ⋯   11 p
      4) Neovascularization   ⋯   12 p
      5) Lipolysis Effect   ⋯   12 p
   5. Types and Characteristics of Threads Used in Thread Embedding Acupuncture
      ⋯   12 p

Ⅱ. Clinical Application of Thread Embedding Acupuncture
   1. Instruments and Preparation
      1) Essential Tools   ⋯   14 p
      2) Pre-treatment Setup   ⋯   16 p
   2. Precautions
      1) Clinical Safety Considerations   ⋯   17 p
      2) Post-Treatment Patient Guidelines   ⋯   18 p
      3) General Safety of Thread Embedding Acupuncture   ⋯   18 p
   3. Physiological Responses After Thread Embedding
      1) Collagen Production Through Thread Absorption   ⋯   19 p

Table of Contents

    2) Foreign Body Reaction (FBR) ⋯ 20 p
    3) Importance of Pre-treatment Patient Disclosure ⋯ 20 p

Ⅲ. Chronic Pain and Thread Embedding Acupuncture
   1. Definition and Classification of Chronic Pain ⋯ 21 p
   2. Limitations of Conventional Treatments and the Role of Thread Embedding Acupuncture
     1) Limitations of Conventional Treatments ⋯ 21 p
     2) Advantages and Role of Thread Embedding Acupuncture ⋯ 21 p
   3. Key Principles of Thread Embedding for Chronic Pain
     1) Importance of Postural Balance and Core Stabilization ⋯ 22 p
     2) Significance of the Cervical Spine in Body Alignment and the Nervous System ⋯ 22 p
     3) Principles of Therapeutic Application ⋯ 22 p
     4) Thread Embedding on Bursal Areas ⋯ 27 p

[Principles of Treatment – Korean Association of Thread Embedding Acupuncture for Pain] ⋯ 28 p

Ⅳ. Clinical Cases and Protocols
   1. Cervical, Thoracic, and Lumbar Spine Regions ⋯ 29 p
   2. Pelvic Region ⋯ 59 p
   3. Knee Joint ⋯ 71 p
   4. Ankle Joint ⋯ 98 p
   5. Shoulder Joint ⋯ 111 p
   6. Elbow Joint ⋯ 130 p
   7. Wrist Joint ⋯ 152 p

Ⅴ. Case Studies ⋯ 164 p

Ⅵ. References ⋯ 165 p

I. Thread Embedding Acupuncture

1. Overview and History of Thread Embedding Acupuncture

Thread Embedding Acupuncture (TEA, Maeseon Ryobeop, 埋線療法) is a treatment modality in which foreign materials are implanted into acupoints, meridians, myofascial lines, or subcutaneous tissue to provide continuous stimulation for therapeutic purposes. While it shares the core mechanisms of traditional acupuncture, thread embedding enhances therapeutic efficacy through prolonged stimulation induced by the physical and biochemical presence of the embedded material.

According to recent trends in clinical research conducted in Korea, Thread Embedding Acupuncture is widely applied in the treatment of musculoskeletal disorders associated with pain, as well as in cosmetic and aesthetic medicine. Its clinical application is expanding into internal medicine, gynecology (e.g., menopausal syndrome), and psychiatry (e.g., depression, neurosis). Particularly in the management of chronic conditions such as patellar dislocation and lumbar disc herniation, Thread Embedding Acupuncture has shown promising outcomes. Expected effects include improvement of nerve function and reflex regulation, enhancement of immune function, better local circulation, suppression of inflammatory mediators, reduction in cellular apoptosis, modulation of cytokine activity, and stimulation of metabolism.

Historically, chromic catgut (羊腸線) was the primary material used for embedding, but in recent years, Polydioxanone (PDO) threads have become the standard. As a monofilament material, PDO is less conducive to bacterial colonization. It retains about 50% of its tensile strength within 3–4 weeks and is mostly absorbed by the body within six months, making it relatively safe. Ongoing research continues to improve the safety and efficacy of thread embedding materials and techniques.

2. Theoretical Foundations of Thread Embedding Acupuncture

1) Relationship Between Meridian Theory and Thread Embedding

Thread Embedding Acupuncture is fundamentally rooted in the meridian theory of Korean medicine. It is based on the interconnectedness of acupoints, meridians, myofascial channels, and cutaneous zones that govern the flow of energy (Qi) and blood throughout the body. Threads are inserted into these strategic anatomical and energetic points—such as acupuncture points and muscular lines—to deliver sustained

I. Thread Embedding Acupuncture

mechanical and biochemical stimulation. This continuous stimulation helps to activate the body's innate healing capacity, restore physiological function, and alleviate chronic pain and dysfunction. Thread Embedding Acupuncture is thus widely applied across various conditions based on theories of cutaneous zones, meridian pathways, and muscle channels.

2) Anatomical Basis for Thread Embedding Acupuncture

Thread embedding therapy involves inserting threads into anatomical connective tissues related to pain, such as fascia, muscles, tendinous sheaths, and ligaments. Thread embedding is also grounded in anatomical precision. Threads are inserted into structures associated with pain, including muscles, ligaments, nerves, and blood vessels. The presence of the thread induces sustained stimulation at the site, enhancing local circulation, promoting tissue regeneration, reducing inflammation, and alleviating pain. It is particularly effective in treating chronic soft tissue injuries and trigger points near nerves, contributing to functional recovery and pain relief. A detailed understanding of anatomy is essential for maximizing both the efficacy and safety of the procedure.

3) Application of Thread Embedding Acupuncture to Trigger Points

Trigger points are hyperirritable nodules located within taut bands of skeletal muscle and are recognized as a common source of chronic musculoskeletal pain. Thread Embedding Acupuncture targets these points by providing prolonged stimulation through implanted threads. This stimulation reduces muscular tension, improves microcirculation, and interrupts pain signaling pathways. Clinical studies suggest that thread embedding may offer longer-lasting therapeutic effects compared to traditional acupuncture when applied to trigger points.

3. Mechanism of Action

As part of the general healing response, thread embedding induces the inflammatory, proliferative, and maturation phases, promoting connective tissue regeneration. This process not only aids in the repair of damaged tissues but also enhances their elasticity and tensile strength.

I. Thread Embedding Acupuncture

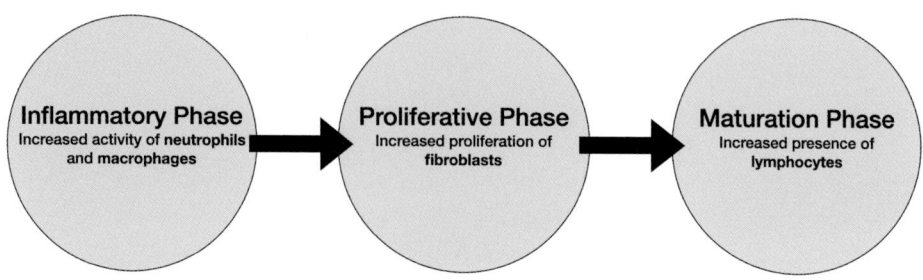

4. Clinical Effects of Thread Embedding Acupuncture

1) Enhanced Function of Muscle Spindles & Golgi Tendon Organs

Thread Embedding Acupuncture involves the insertion of specialized threads into muscle tissue, providing continuous stimulation that activates mechanoreceptors such as muscle spindles and Golgi tendon organs. This sustained stimulation helps regulate muscle tone and enhances neuromuscular feedback, which has been shown to contribute positively to the alleviation of chronic musculoskeletal pain and the restoration of motor function. Several randomized controlled trials have demonstrated that thread embedding yields superior outcomes in reducing muscle tension and pain compared to traditional acupuncture.

2) Fusimotor Reflex

Thread embedding stimulates intrafusal fibers, thereby activating the fusimotor reflex. This reflex enhances the sensitivity of sensory nerves within muscles, facilitating fine motor control and modulation of muscle tone. Clinically, patients have reported reduced muscle stiffness and improved range of motion following thread embedding, suggesting that activation of the fusimotor reflex is one of the key mechanisms contributing to therapeutic effectiveness.

3) Collagen Regeneration

The continuous mechanical stimulation from embedded threads induces controlled micro-injury and localized inflammatory responses, which in turn activate fibroblasts and promote collagen regeneration. In facial rejuvenation studies, thread embedding has been shown to significantly reduce wrinkle depth and area while improving skin elasticity. These effects are attributed to collagen synthesis and restructuring of the dermal matrix.

I. Thread Embedding Acupuncture

4) Neovascularization

Thread embedding improves local blood flow and promotes neovascularization (formation of new blood vessels). The localized microtrauma and inflammation caused by thread insertion stimulate the expression of angiogenic factors such as vascular endothelial growth factor (VEGF). Clinically, this mechanism is associated with enhanced tissue regeneration and skin rejuvenation effects.

5) Lipolysis Effect

In the field of obesity treatment, thread embedding has been observed to facilitate lipid metabolism and promote lipolysis (breakdown of fat cells). Continuous stimulation from the inserted threads improves microcirculation and activates metabolic processes within adipocytes. Clinical studies have reported reductions in abdominal circumference and subcutaneous fat thickness, supporting the interpretation that improved local circulation and stimulated lipolysis underlie these outcomes.

5. Types and Characteristics of Threads Used in Thread Embedding Acupuncture

The materials used for thread embedding vary depending on the therapeutic purpose and the anatomical target area. The most commonly used types include the following:

Types of Threads	Characteristics, Advantages, and Disadvantages
PDO (Polydioxanone)	A biodegradable synthetic polymer that is fully absorbed by the body within 6 months to 1 year. It causes minimal tissue irritation and is considered highly safe, making it the most widely used material in Thread Embedding Acupuncture. Its relatively fast absorption allows for easy repeat procedures.

I. Thread Embedding Acupuncture

Types of Threads	Characteristics, Advantages, and Disadvantages
PLLA (Poly-L-lactic acid)	A biodegradable polymer that decomposes slowly in the body, providing long-lasting stimulation for 1 to 2 years. It is highly effective in promoting collagen regeneration, making it widely used in aesthetic and dermatological applications. However, rare side effects such as nodule formation have been reported.
PLCL (Poly-L-lactide-co-ε-caprolactone)	A composite material that combines the properties of PLLA and PCL, offering a moderate degradation rate with excellent elasticity and stimulatory effects. It provides sustained tissue stimulation over a relatively long period.

All of these threads are naturally biodegradable within the body and induce a range of physiological effects, including tissue regeneration, collagen production, and improved blood circulation.

The duration of stimulation, tissue response, and safety profile vary depending on the material used, so thread selection should be tailored to the patient's condition and the therapeutic goals.

II. Clinical Application of Thread Embedding Acupuncture

1. Instruments and Preparation

1) Essential Tools
   ① Thread Needle
   · A needle device preloaded with a specialized thread (e.g., PDO, PLLA), available in various lengths and thicknesses depending on the treatment area.
   · Single-use, pre-sterilized needles are used to minimize the risk of infection.
   · Miracu Plus – Manufactured by Dongbang Medical Co., Ltd. (Republic of Korea).

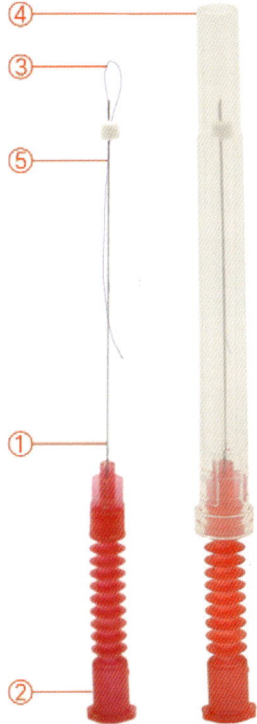

Miracu Plus

This product features a flexible hub, allowing for easy manipulation from various angles during treatment. It is designed for convenience, precision, and safety in thread embedding procedures. This product is patented. (Korean Patent Application No. 10-2016-0088483).

Its components include:

II. Clinical Application of Thread Embedding Acupuncture

❶ Needle Cannula (침관, Chim-gwan) : The portion inserted into the body, used for delivering the absorbable thread.
❷ Hub (침기, Chim-gi) : The handle-like part that secures the cannula and facilitates easy attachment and manipulation during the procedure.
❸ Biodegradable Absorbable Thread (PDO : Polydioxanone) : The absorbable thread implanted into the muscle tissue.
❹ Protective Cap : Covers the needle and thread to protect them during storage.
❺ Sponge : Holds the thread and cannula in place when the protective cap is removed, preventing accidental separation.

As shown in the image below, Miracu Plus can also be connected to a syringe to allow simultaneous administration of pharmacopuncture alongside Thread Embedding Acupuncture.

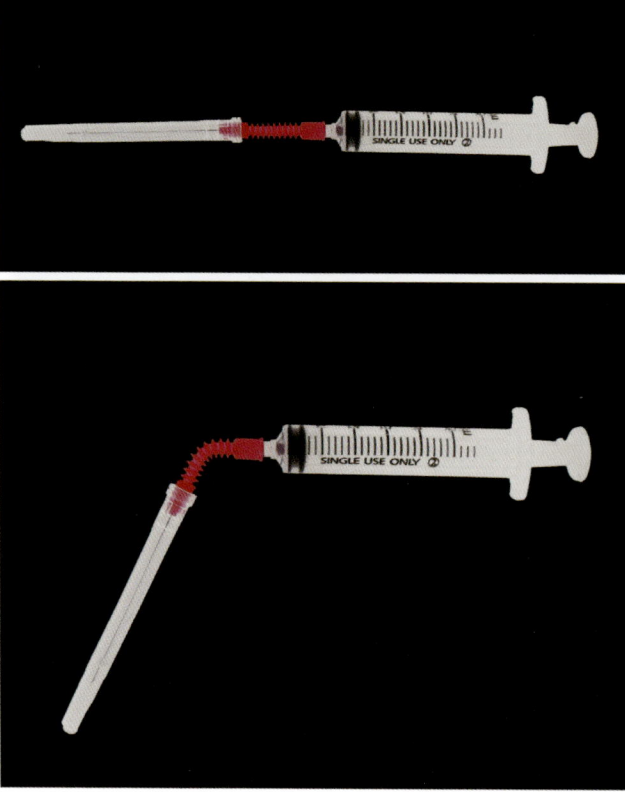

II. Clinical Application of Thread Embedding Acupuncture

② Disinfection Supplies

To prevent infection at the treatment site, essential disinfection items such as alcohol swabs, antiseptic solution, and sterile gauze must be prepared.

Both the instruments and the treatment area must be thoroughly sterilized before and after the procedure.

③ Topical Anesthetic Cream

For patients with high pain sensitivity or in cases involving specialized threads, a topical anesthetic cream may be applied for 15–30 minutes.

General thread needles can typically be used without anesthesia, but the use of anesthetic cream can be considered based on the patient's condition.

④ Cold Compress Tools

Cold packs should be prepared to reduce bruising, swelling, and discomfort after treatment.

Apply for 10–15 minutes post-procedure to promote recovery.

2) Pre-treatment Setup

- Patient Consultation & Treatment Planning: Determine the treatment area based on the patient's condition and treatment goals.
- Consent Form & Pre-treatment Photography: Obtain informed consent and record baseline photos prior to treatment.
- Sterilization of Treatment Area: Thorough disinfection is performed to prevent infection.
- Application of Anesthetic Cream (if needed): Apply to the treatment site and allow sufficient absorption time.
- Thread Needle Preparation: Use single-use, sterile thread needles only.
- Post-Treatment Care & Instructions: Apply a hot compress to reduce bruising and swelling, and provide aftercare guidance to support healing.

II. Clinical Application of Thread Embedding Acupuncture

2. Precautions

1) Clinical Safety Considerations

　① Do Not Reinsert the Needle After Withdrawal

　Unlike general acupuncture or pharmacopuncture, thread embedding must not involve withdrawing and reinserting the needle when encountering anatomical structures such as bone, blood vessels, or nerves.

　Reinsertion can cause the embedded thread to twist or tangle within the tissue, leading to serious complications such as chronic inflammation, foreign body sensation, or tissue damage.

　To prevent these issues, an accurate understanding of anatomical structures is essential, and the needle insertion direction must be precisely determined from the outset using the other hand."

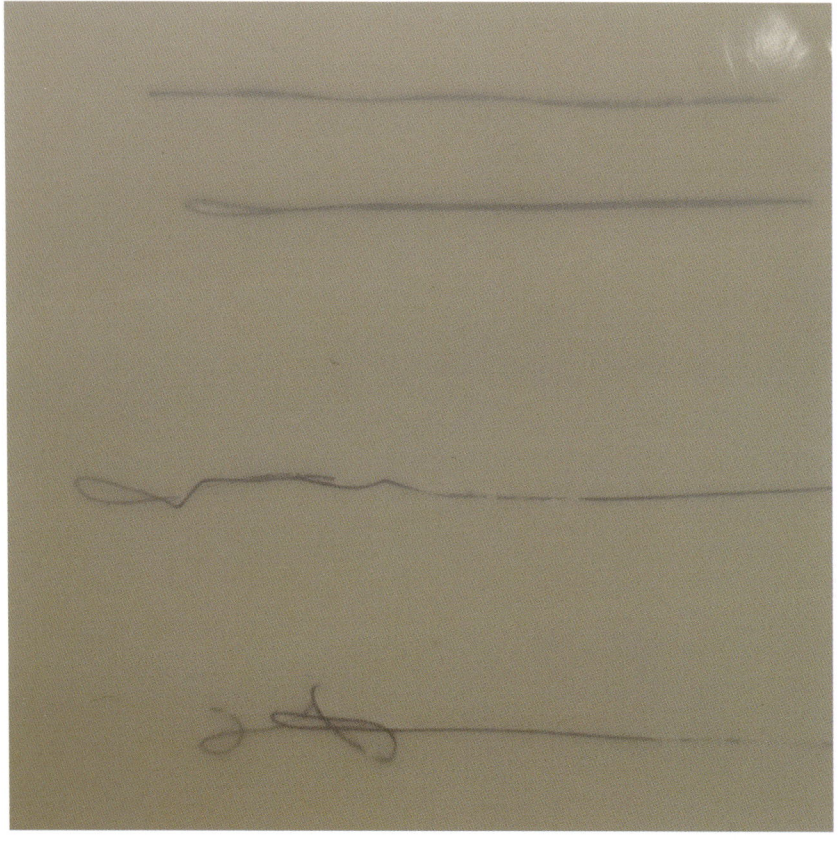

II. Clinical Application of Thread Embedding Acupuncture

(Photographic example using a practice model: The first and second threads were inserted in a straight line, while the third and fourth threads demonstrate entanglement due to withdrawal and reinsertion, clearly showing the risks of improper technique.)

② Needle Removal After Thread Insertion

After inserting the thread, gently rotate the hub of the needle 3 to 5 times to help the thread adhere to the surrounding tissue.

Then, while lightly pressing on the skin with a support finger, slowly and steadily withdraw the needle to complete the procedure.

③ Management of Threads Protruding from the Skin

Occasionally, part of the thread may remain exposed outside the skin after insertion. In such cases, the following stepwise approach is recommended:

- If only a small portion of the thread remains visible, gently stretch the surrounding skin to help guide the thread naturally into the body.
- If the thread does not fully retract, use sterilized surgical scissors to trim the exposed portion. To prevent infection, ensure the scissors are thoroughly disinfected, and use both blades to gently press the skin so that the thread can be cut as close to the skin surface as possible.
- The safest and most effective method is to remove the exposed thread entirely and reinsert a new thread at the appropriate site. This approach minimizes the risk of infection, foreign body reaction, and skin irritation.

2) Post-Treatment Patient Guidelines

Patients should avoid alcohol consumption and strong external stimuli—such as massage, sauna, or radiofrequency therapy—for at least one week following the procedure.

Temporary bruising, swelling, a foreign body sensation, or mild discomfort at the insertion site may occur, but these symptoms typically subside within 1 to 2 weeks.

3) General Safety of Thread Embedding Acupuncture

Thread Embedding Acupuncture is generally considered a safe procedure; however, several precautions should be observed:

- Possible side effects include localized infection, bleeding, bruising, and, in rare

II. Clinical Application of Thread Embedding Acupuncture

cases, nerve damage.
- Strict adherence to aseptic protocols and performance by a well-trained practitioner are essential.
- Patients taking anticoagulants, those with bleeding disorders, pregnant women, dialysis patients, insulin users, and those on thyroid medications must consult a medical specialist before undergoing the procedure.

Although research on the efficacy and safety of Thread Embedding Acupuncture (TEA) is accumulating, large-scale randomized controlled trials (RCTs) are still needed.

For example, a pilot RCT by Lee (2018) evaluated the efficacy and safety of TEA for patients with chronic low back pain. A total of 40 participants were enrolled: the TEA group (experimental group) received four TEA sessions at 2-week intervals over 8 weeks, while the control group received conventional acupuncture twice a week for a total of 16 sessions.

The primary outcome was the Visual Analog Scale (VAS) for pain, with secondary outcomes including the Short-Form McGill Pain Questionnaire (SF-MPQ) and Oswestry Disability Index (ODI).

Both groups showed significant improvement in pain and function over time; however, the TEA group demonstrated notably greater improvement in ODI scores. No serious adverse events were reported during the study, supporting the potential safety and effectiveness of TEA and providing foundational data for future large-scale clinical trials.

3. Physiological Responses After Thread Embedding

1) Collagen Production Through Thread Absorption

Absorbable threads used in Thread Embedding Acupuncture—such as PDO, PLLA, and PCL—gradually degrade and are absorbed by the body over time. During this process, surrounding tissues often exhibit enhanced collagen production.

For example, PCL threads are completely absorbed over 12 to 18 months. Animal studies have shown increased expression of new collagen, type III collagen, and transforming growth factor-beta (TGF-β) during this period.

Similarly, in animal models using PDO threads, significant tissue responses were

II. Clinical Application of Thread Embedding Acupuncture

observed over 24 weeks, including collagen synthesis, formation of new fibrous connective tissue, fat reduction, tissue contraction, and improved vascularization.
These physiological changes are closely linked to the aesthetic benefits of Thread Embedding Acupuncture, such as skin regeneration and wrinkle reduction.

2) Foreign Body Reaction (FBR)
When any foreign material, including thread, is introduced into the body, a foreign body reaction is inevitable. This begins with acute inflammation immediately following insertion and may progress to chronic inflammation and fibrosis over weeks or months. During this process, immune cells such as macrophages gather around the thread to either break it down or encapsulate it.

However, in some cases, the body may not fully absorb the thread and may attempt to expel it. This can result in thread extrusion through the insertion point—or, rarely, through mucosal surfaces such as the eyes or mouth—several days to weeks after the procedure.

Clinically, complications have been reported such as thread exposure, protrusion, localized infection, inflammation, or skin depression when threads fail to degrade properly.

Common causes of thread extrusion include:
- Insertion too close to the surface of the skin
- Use of excessively long or thick threads
- Poor local blood circulation
- Inadequate insertion technique or practitioner inexperience

3) Importance of Pre-Treatment Patient Disclosure
Prior to the procedure, it is essential to inform patients that while threads are intended to be absorbed and stimulate collagen production, foreign body reactions may lead to thread extrusion in rare cases.

Patients must be clearly advised about the potential risks—including thread exposure, protrusion, infection, and inflammation—and instructed on what to do if such complications occur.

Proper consent and education help manage expectations and ensure timely intervention when needed.

III. Chronic Pain and Thread Embedding Acupuncture

1. Definition and Classification of Chronic Pain

Chronic pain is generally defined as pain that persists for more than 3 to 6 months, or pain that continues even after tissue healing has occurred.
According to the International Association for the Study of Pain (IASP), chronic pain is "pain that persists beyond the expected period of healing following an acute illness or injury" and is recognized not merely as a symptom, but as a distinct clinical condition.

Chronic pain is typically classified as follows:
- Neuropathic Pain: Arising from damage or dysfunction of the nervous system, characterized by burning sensations, allodynia, and hyperalgesia.
- Musculoskeletal Pain: Originating from structural damage or diseases affecting bones, muscles, joints, or ligaments. Common examples include chronic low back pain, arthritis, and fibromyalgia.
- Inflammatory Pain: Caused by tissue injury and inflammatory processes, as seen in conditions like rheumatoid arthritis.
- Functional Pain: Occurs without structural damage but due to abnormal neural responses or altered nervous system function, including fibromyalgia and irritable bowel syndrome.

2. Limitations of Conventional Treatments and the Role of Thread Embedding Acupuncture

1) Limitations of Conventional Treatments

Chronic pain management often involves medications (analgesics, antidepressants, anticonvulsants), physical therapy, psychological interventions, injection therapy, and nerve blocks.
However, these approaches frequently fall short due to side effects, tolerance development, and incomplete symptom relief. Moreover, a strictly pathoanatomical approach may not adequately address the complex, multifactorial nature of chronic pain.

2) Advantages and Role of Thread Embedding Acupuncture
- Fewer side effects compared to pharmacologic treatment
- No risk of drug dependence

III. Chronic Pain and Thread Embedding Acupuncture

- Repeatable procedures with potential long-term effects in some patients
- An effective complementary or alternative option for patients with treatment-resistant chronic pain
- Effective in treating chronic pain by addressing musculoskeletal structural instability

3. Key Principles of Thread Embedding for Chronic Pain

1) Importance of Postural Balance and Core Stabilization

Core stability plays a crucial role in maintaining the biomechanical integrity of the spine-pelvis complex and enhancing neuromuscular control in patients with chronic pain such as low back pain.

Activation of core muscles—such as the transversus abdominis, multifidus, and obliques—supports spinal stability, reduces joint overload, and prevents muscle fatigue. Numerous studies have shown that core stabilization improves pain levels, physical function, muscle thickness, and strength.

For example:
- The psoas major is essential for lumbar lordosis and hip flexion; dysfunction is strongly linked to low back pain.
- The gluteus medius is responsible for hip abduction and pelvic stability during gait; its weakness is associated with a positive Trendelenburg sign.

2) Significance of the Cervical Spine in Body Alignment and the Nervous System

Cervical alignment significantly affects overall body posture and central nervous system function.

Stabilizing the cervical spine can reduce pain, improve function, and correct postural imbalances—particularly forward head posture.

Cervical muscle activation and postural correction are linked to neurophysiological functions such as motor control, balance, and modulation of lower extremity tone via vestibulospinal pathways.

3) Principles of Therapeutic Application

Thread Embedding Acupuncture(PDO) involves inserting absorbable threads into muscles or fascia, where they provide sustained mechanical and biochemical stimulation.

III. Chronic Pain and Thread Embedding Acupuncture

This induces localized inflammatory responses, promoting tissue regeneration and neuromuscular coordination.

In patients with chronic pain, targeting core muscles (e.g., multifidus, erector spinae, quadratus lumborum, psoas major) and cervical stabilizers with thread insertion can restore trunk stability and reduce pain. An example of Dr. Byung-il Choi's core muscle thread embedding treatment described in Lee (2018) is as follows.

Table 2 Treatment sites for thread-embedding acupuncture in the dorsal area of the human body

	Localization		Direction of insertion	Needle length	Number of pieces inserted
	Muscle	Skeleton			
①	Intrinsic muscle (spinalis, rotatores)	L3–4, L4–5, L5–S1	Perpendicular insertion	40 mm	6 pieces
②	Multifidus muscle	L4–5	Oblique insertion	60 mm	2 pieces
③	Lumbar erector spinae	Sacrum–L5, L3–L1	Transverse insertion	60 mm	4 pieces
④	Iliolumbar ligament	L5–iliac crest	Oblique insertion	60 mm	2 pieces
⑤	Sacroiliac ligament	Posterior inferior iliac spine–coccyx	Oblique insertion	60 mm	2 pieces
⑥	Gluteus medius	–	Transverse insertion	40 mm	2 pieces
⑦	Piriformis	–	Perpendicular insertion	60 mm	2 pieces
⑧	Thoracic vertebrae erector spinae	T7–10	Transverse insertion	60 mm	2 pieces
⑨	Thoracic vertebrae erector spinae	T3–5	Transverse insertion	60 mm	2 pieces
⑩	Trapezius, levator scapulae	C7	Transverse insertion	60 mm	2 pieces
⑪	Cervical vertebrae erector spinae	C4–7	Transverse insertion	40 mm	2 pieces
Total					28 pieces

III. Chronic Pain and Thread Embedding Acupuncture

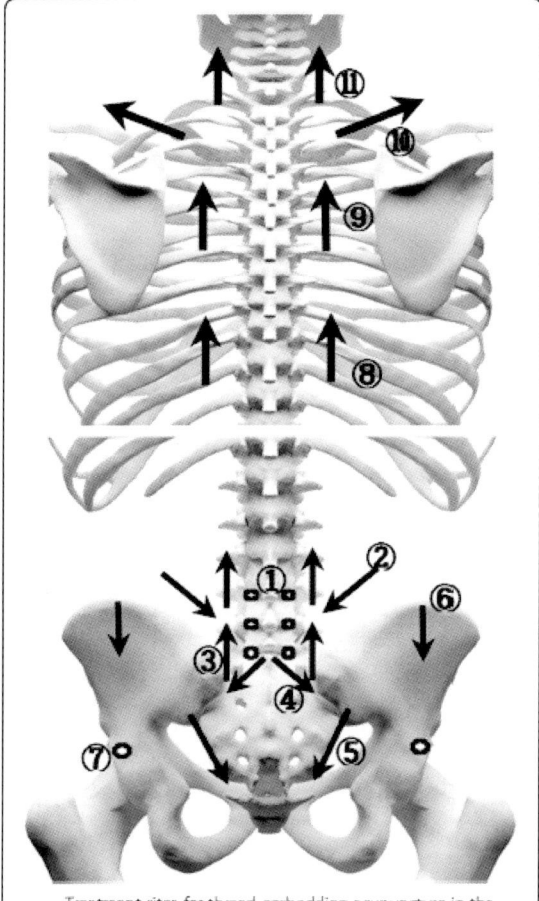

Treatment sites for thread-embedding acupuncture in the dorsal area of the human body

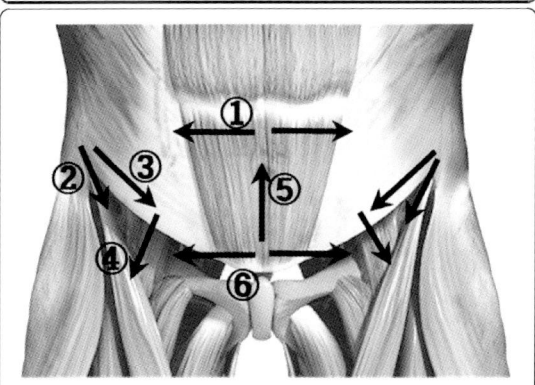

Treatment sites for thread-embedding acupuncture in the abdominal area of the human body

III. Chronic Pain and Thread Embedding Acupuncture

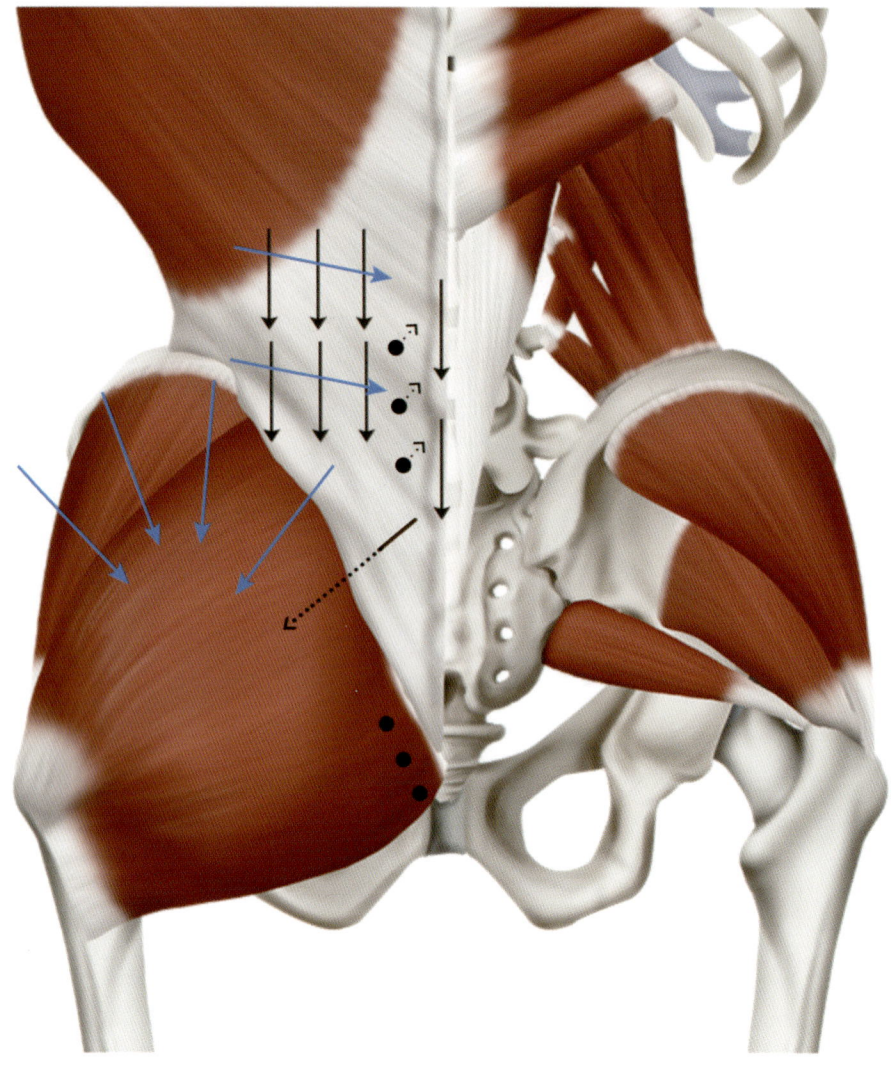

III. Chronic Pain and Thread Embedding Acupuncture

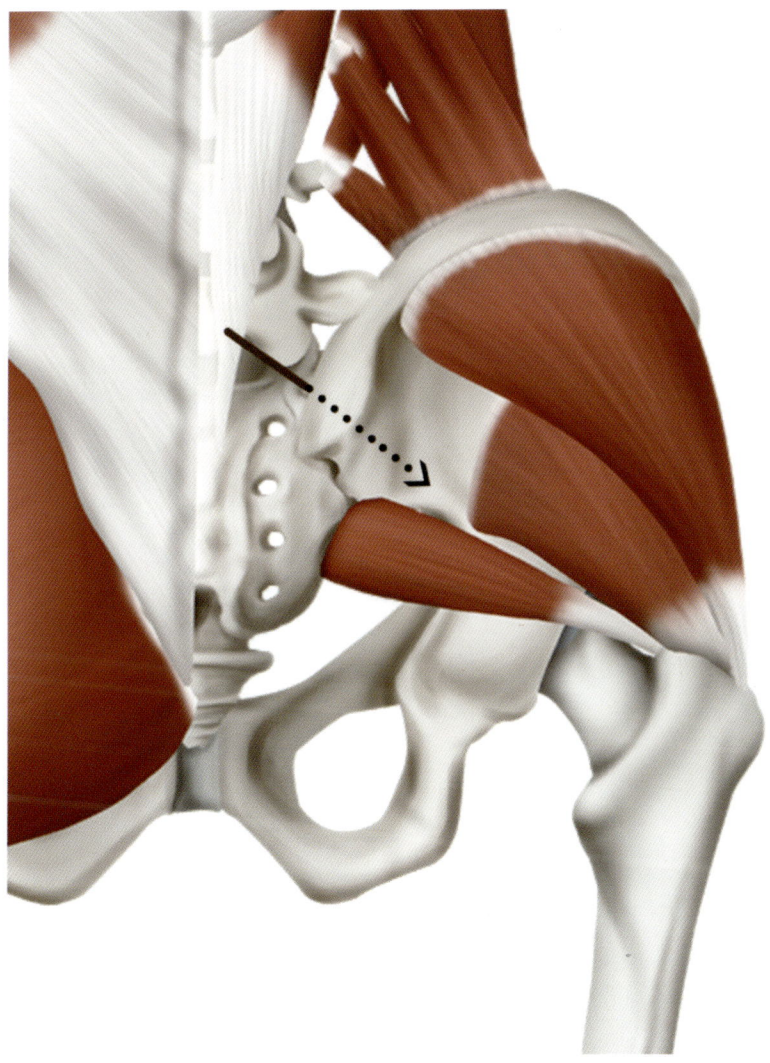

III. Chronic Pain and Thread Embedding Acupuncture

4) Thread Embedding on Bursal Areas

Bursae are small, fluid-filled sacs located around joints, acting as cushions that reduce friction between bones, muscles, tendons, and skin. These structures are especially abundant in frequently moving joints such as the shoulder, knee, and elbow, allowing smooth joint movement.

| Bursitis by anatomical site |

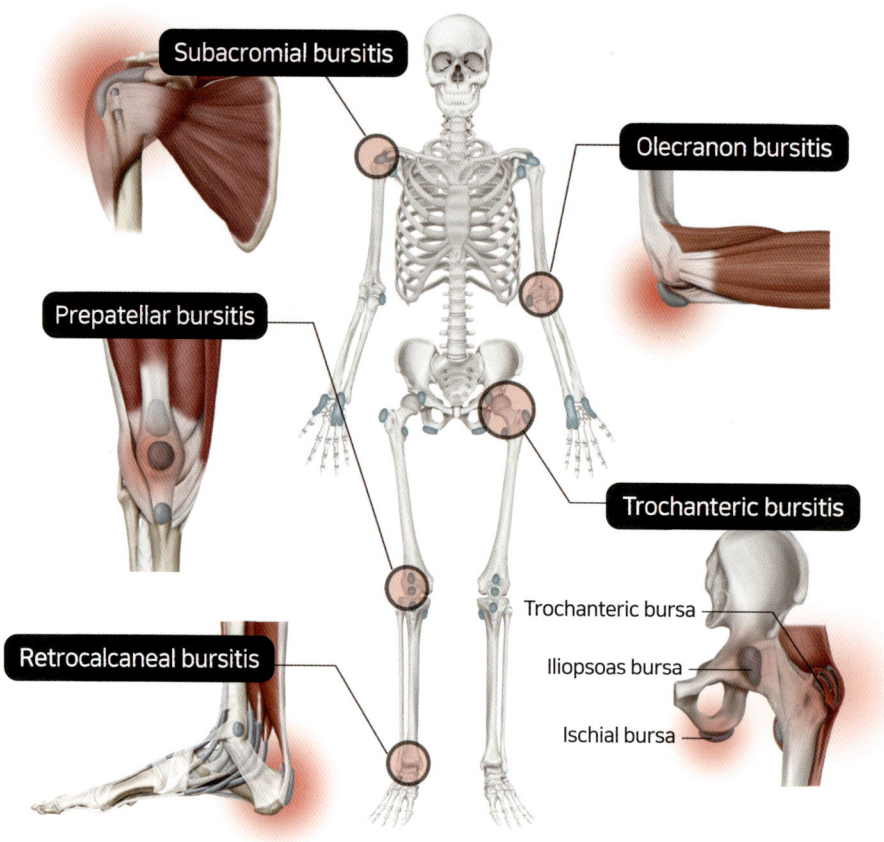

III. Chronic Pain and Thread Embedding Acupuncture

Thread Embedding Acupuncture is particularly effective when applied directly over bursa regions. Chronic bursitis and related peri-bursal pain are often exacerbated by impaired microcirculation, reduced tissue regeneration, and tension in the fascia and surrounding musculature. By inserting threads into the soft tissue surrounding the bursa, continuous mechanical stimulation and mild inflammatory responses are induced, which in turn enhance local blood flow and promote tissue repair.

Studies have reported increased perfusion, pain reduction, and tissue regeneration in areas treated with thread embedding. Additionally, the therapy helps to relieve tension in adjacent muscles and fascia, reducing mechanical pressure and friction on the bursa itself. This contributes to breaking the cycle of chronic pain and inflammation associated with persistent bursitis.

[Principles of Treatment - Korean Association of Thread Embedding Acupuncture for Pain]

1. Use a sufficient quantity of threads in a single session (more than 100 threads possible).
2. Inform the patient in advance that for about 3 to 7 days after the procedure, they may experience a foreign body sensation, pain, or discomfort, and that in very rare cases, the thread may be pushed out of the body.
3. Combine with pharmacopuncture treatment to aid hydrolysis and provide moisture to soft tissues.
4. Considering tissue response, recovery, and minimization of side effects, perform thread embedding once every 2 to 3 weeks, and up to 10 or more sessions depending on symptom severity.
5. Supplement the treatment with weekly patient monitoring and pharmacopuncture or acupuncture sessions one to two times per week.

IV. Clinical Cases and Protocols

1. Cervical, Thoracic, and Lumbar Spine Regions

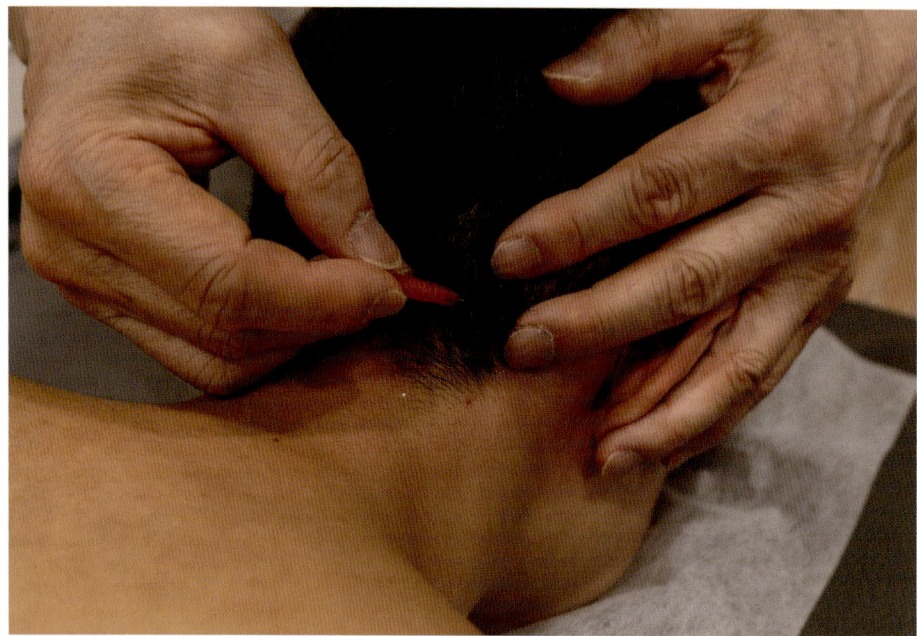

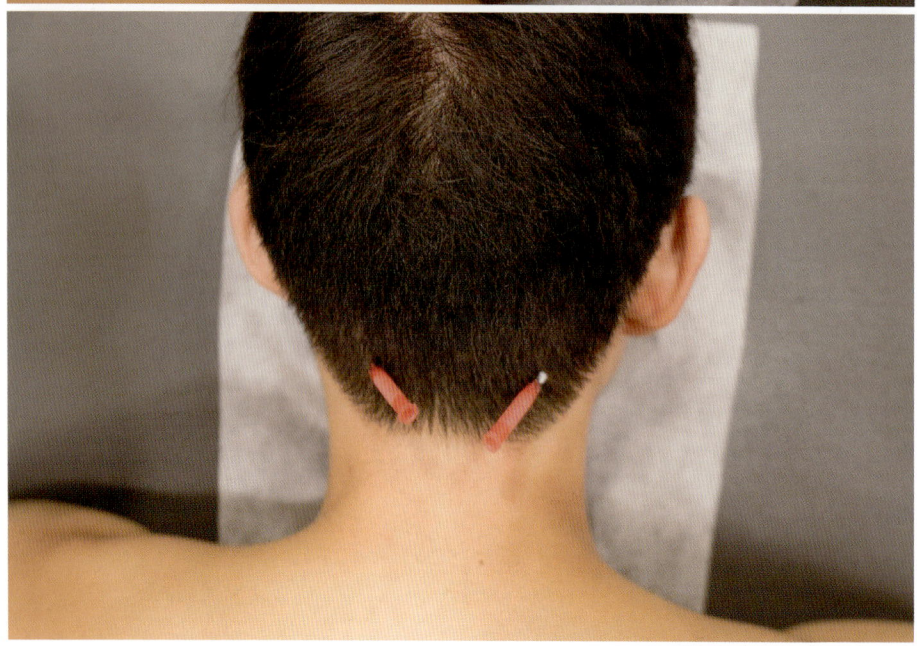

IV. Clinical Cases and Protocols

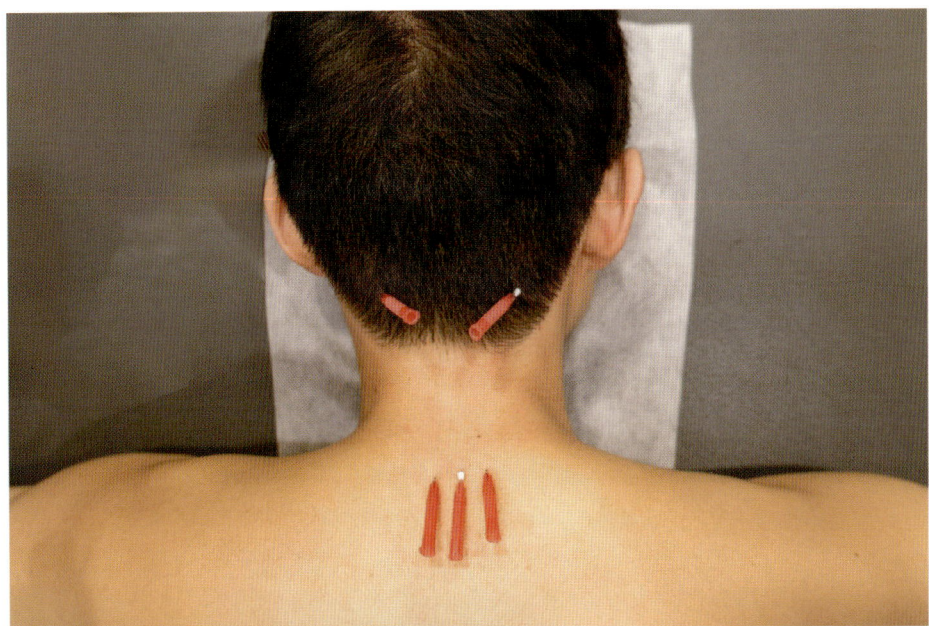

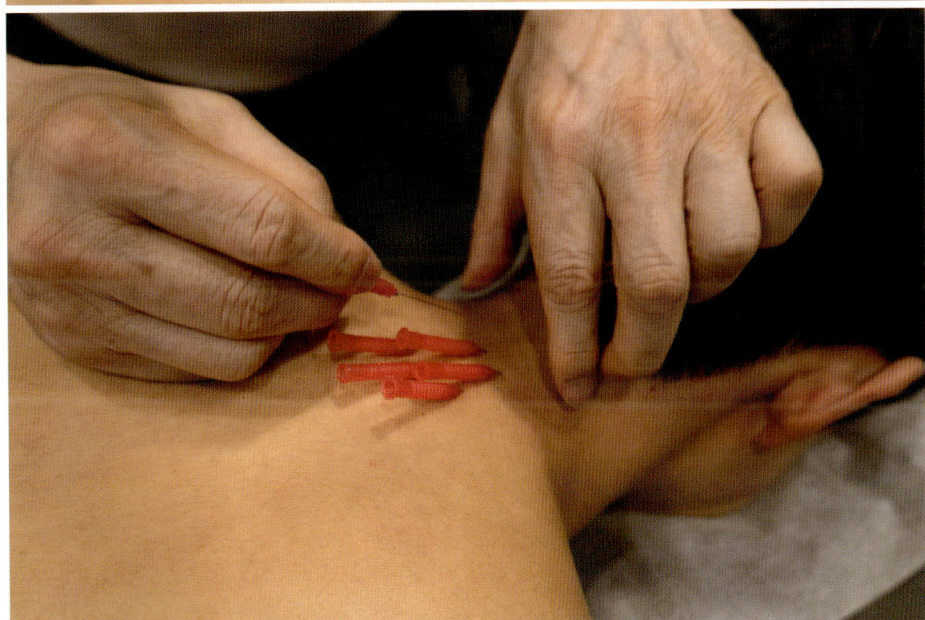

Insert threads transversely into the suboccipital muscles, upper trapezius, and the cervical portion of the erector spinae muscle group—particularly the longissimus muscle, which corresponds to the first line of the Bladder Meridian (Bladder Meridian Line 1).

IV. Clinical Cases and Protocols

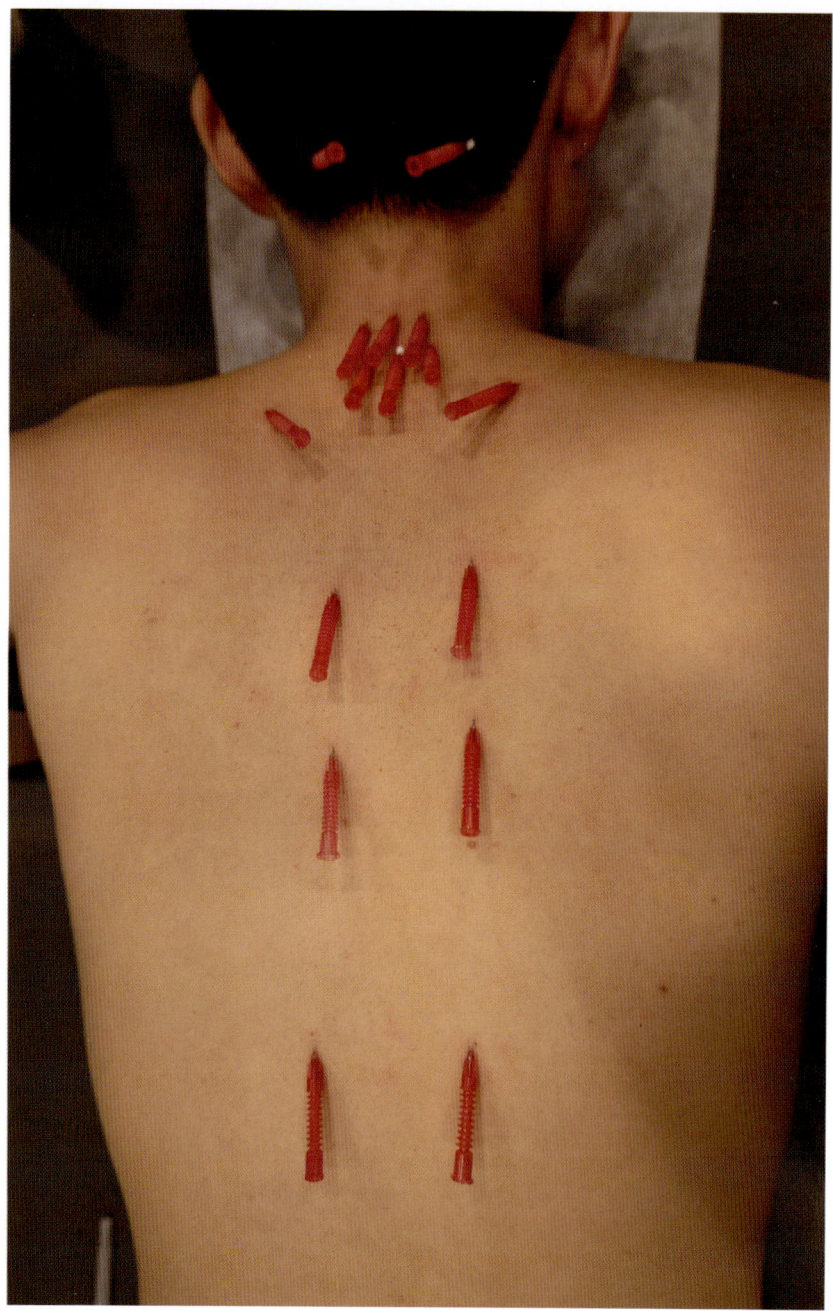

31

IV. Clinical Cases and Protocols

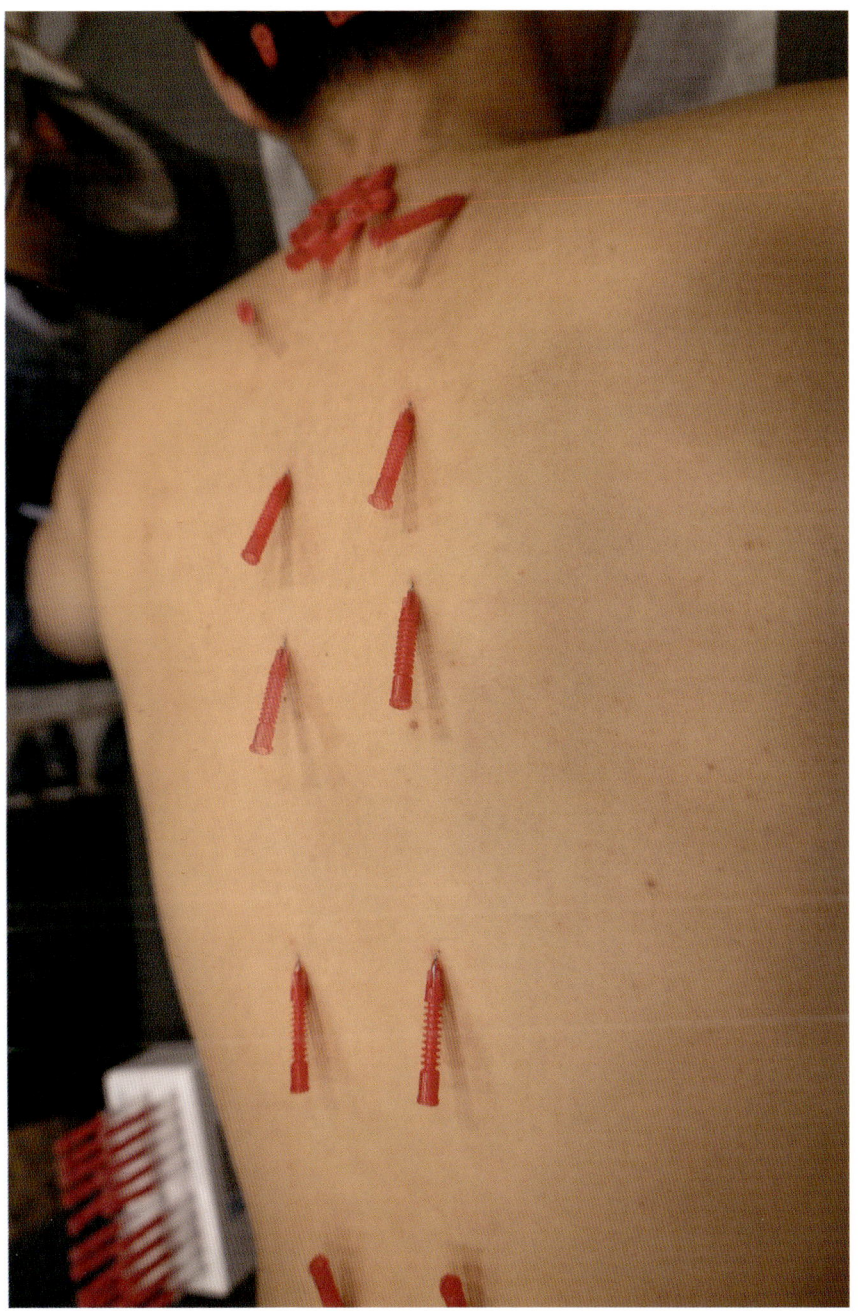

Insert the threads transversely toward the patient's head, targeting the longissimus muscle within the erector spinae group surrounding the thoracic spine.

IV. Clinical Cases and Protocols

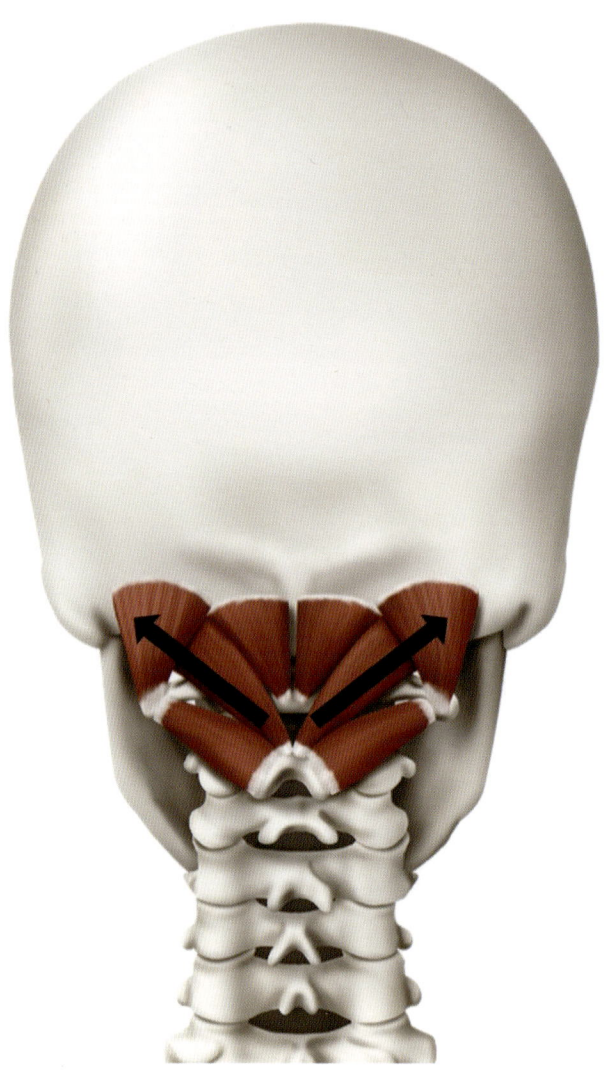

IV. Clinical Cases and Protocols

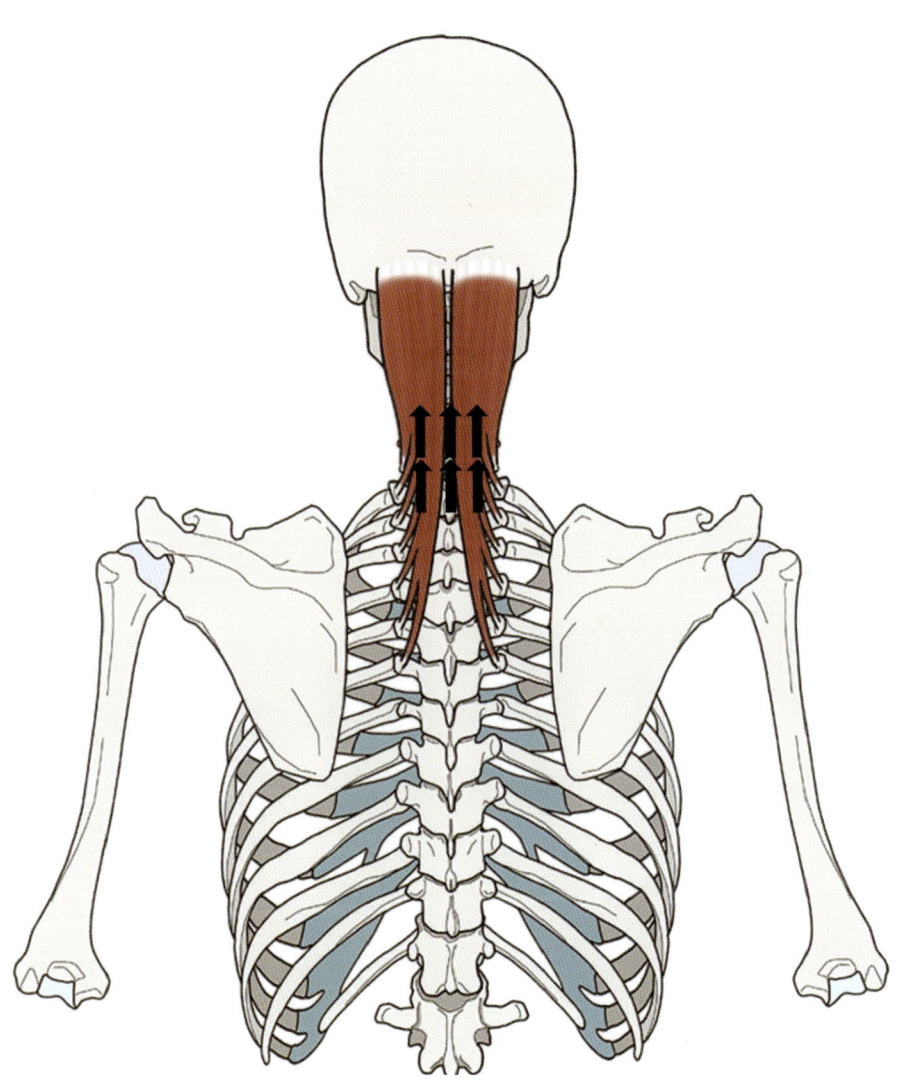

IV. Clinical Cases and Protocols

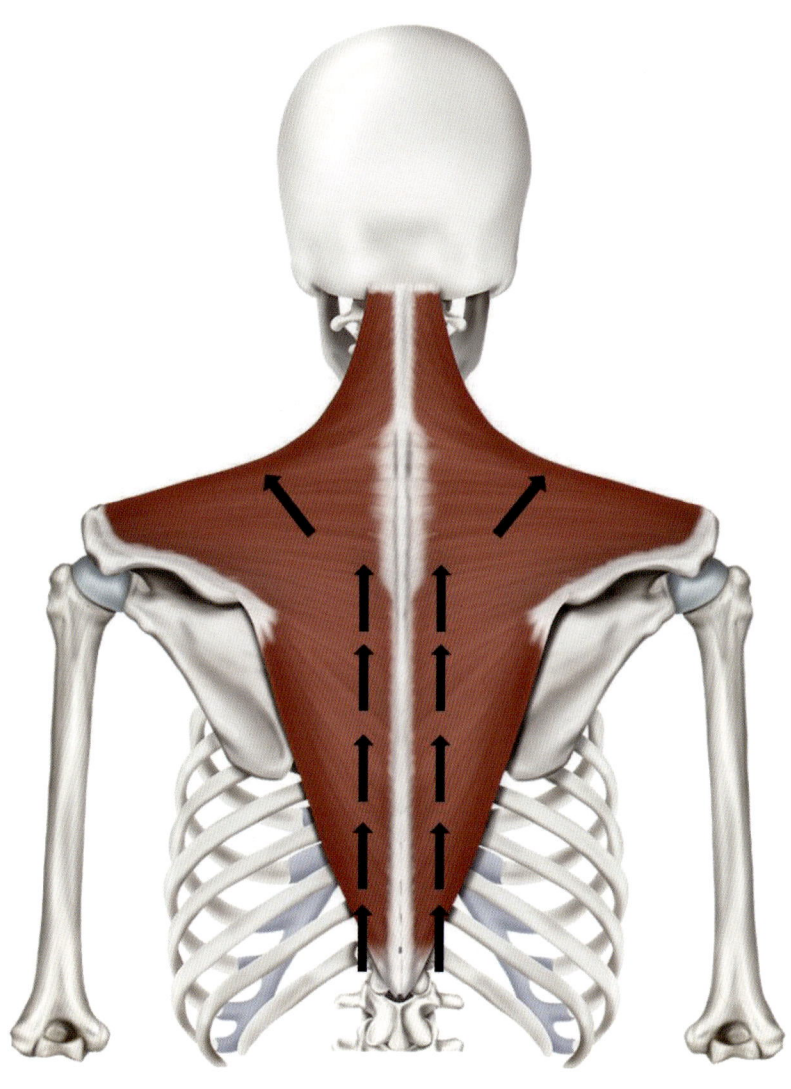

IV. Clinical Cases and Protocols

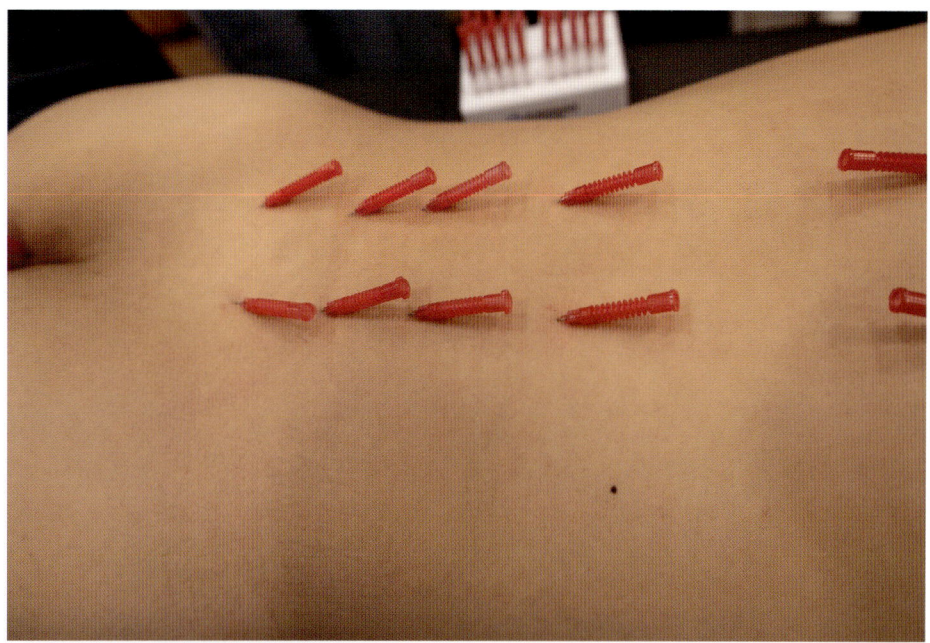

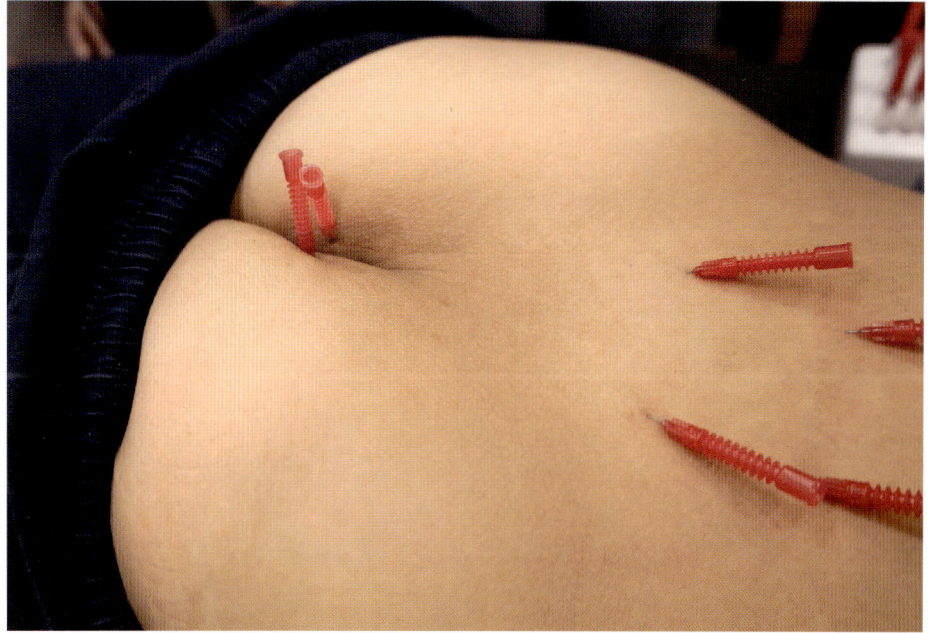

IV. Clinical Cases and Protocols

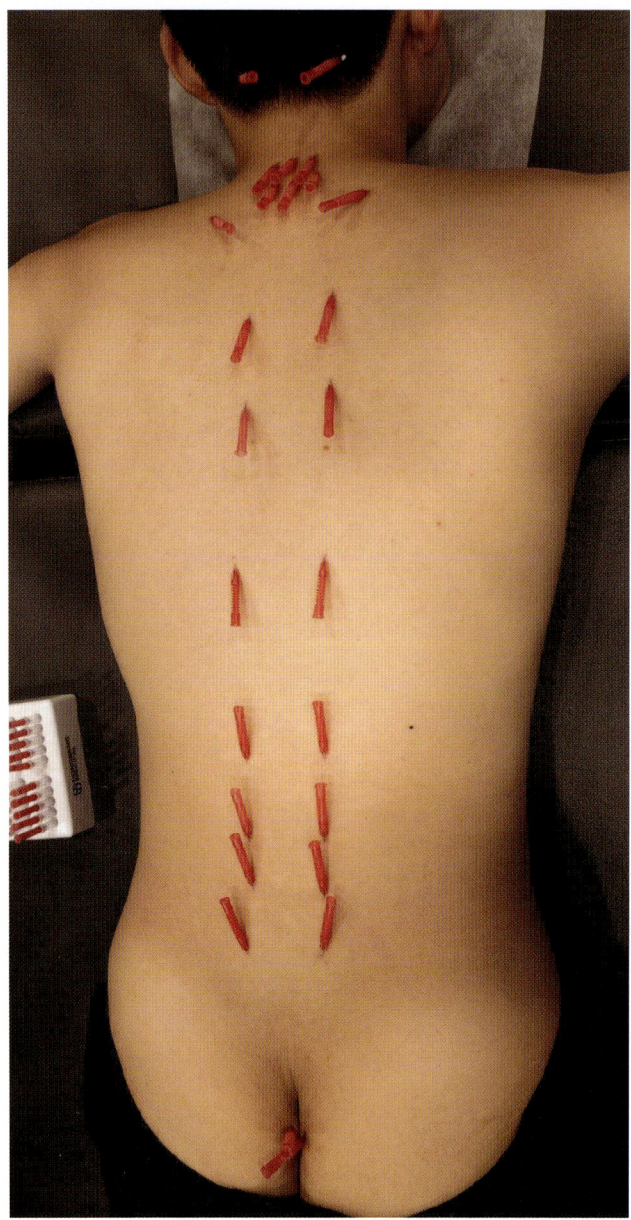

Insert threads transversely toward the patient's head up to the 12th thoracic vertebra (T12), and toward the patient's feet below that level.

Palpate the coccyx, then insert the thread either perpendicularly or obliquely into the coccygeus muscle, close to the bone.

IV. Clinical Cases and Protocols

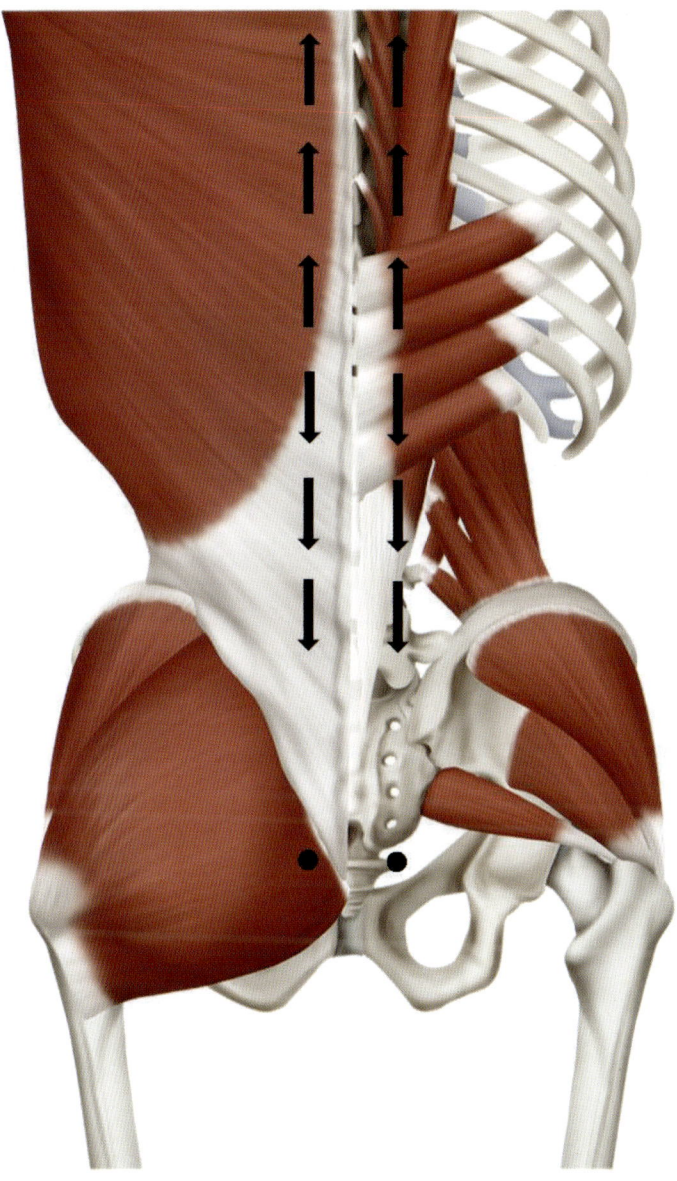

IV. Clinical Cases and Protocols

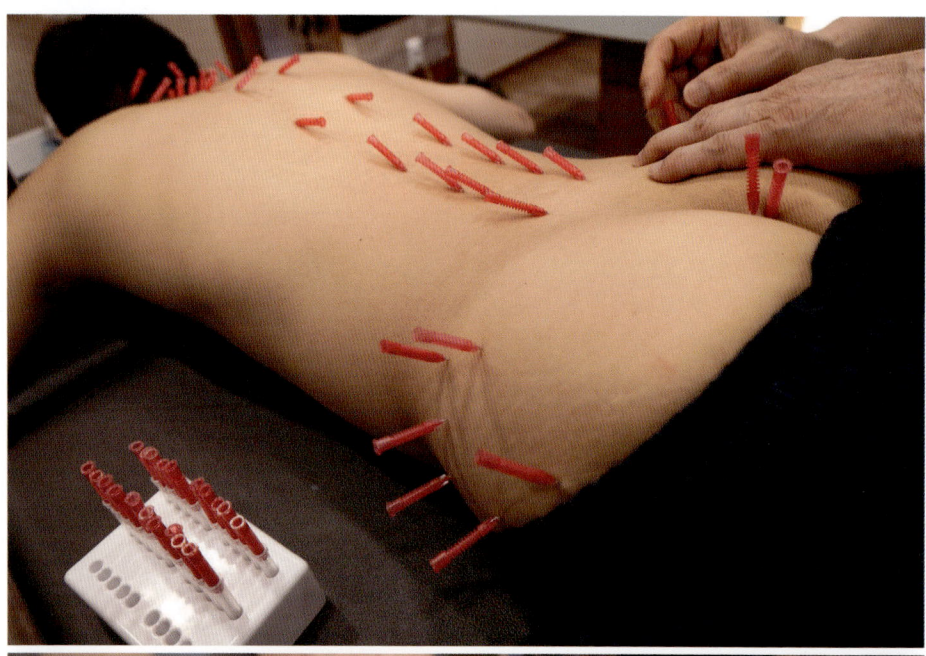

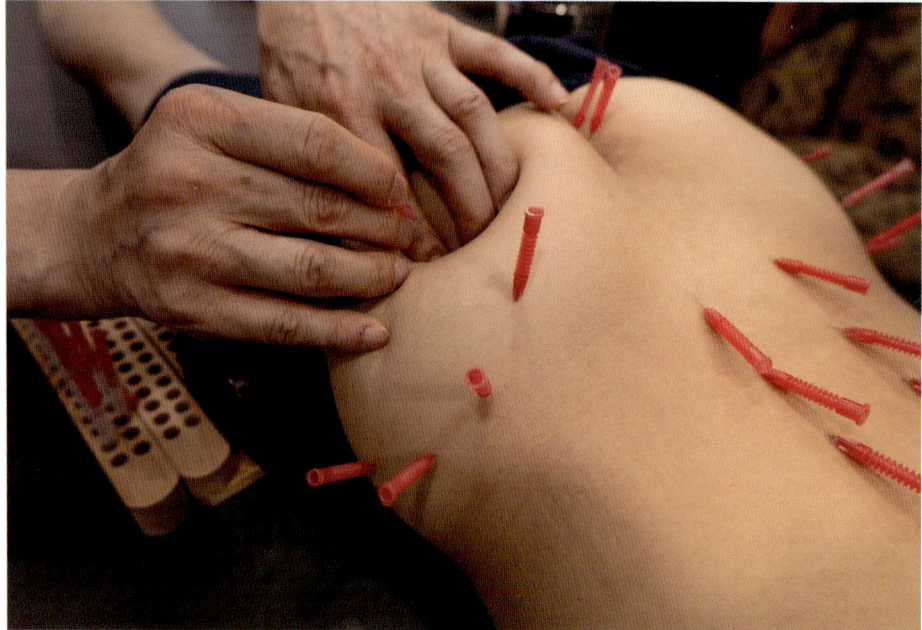

IV. Clinical Cases and Protocols

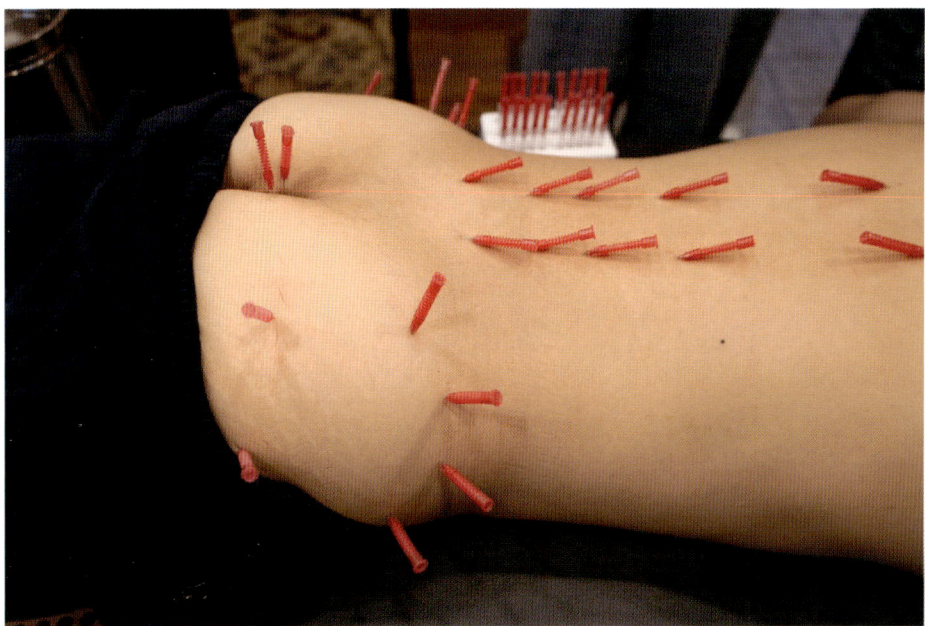

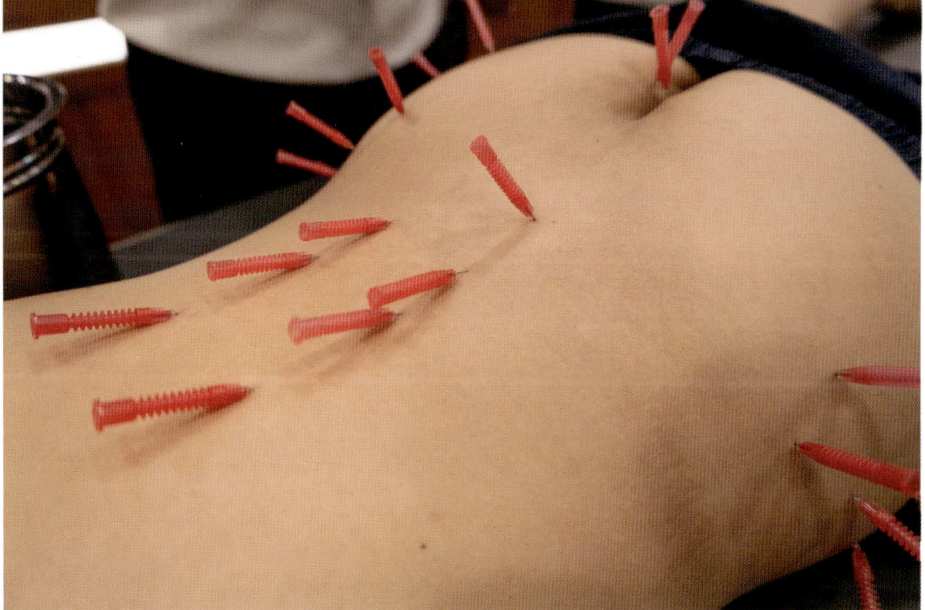

Insert threads obliquely targeting the gluteus maximus, medius, and minimus muscles. For the muscles surrounding the hip joint—such as those near Huan-do (環跳, GB30) and the piriformis muscle—use perpendicular insertion.

IV. Clinical Cases and Protocols

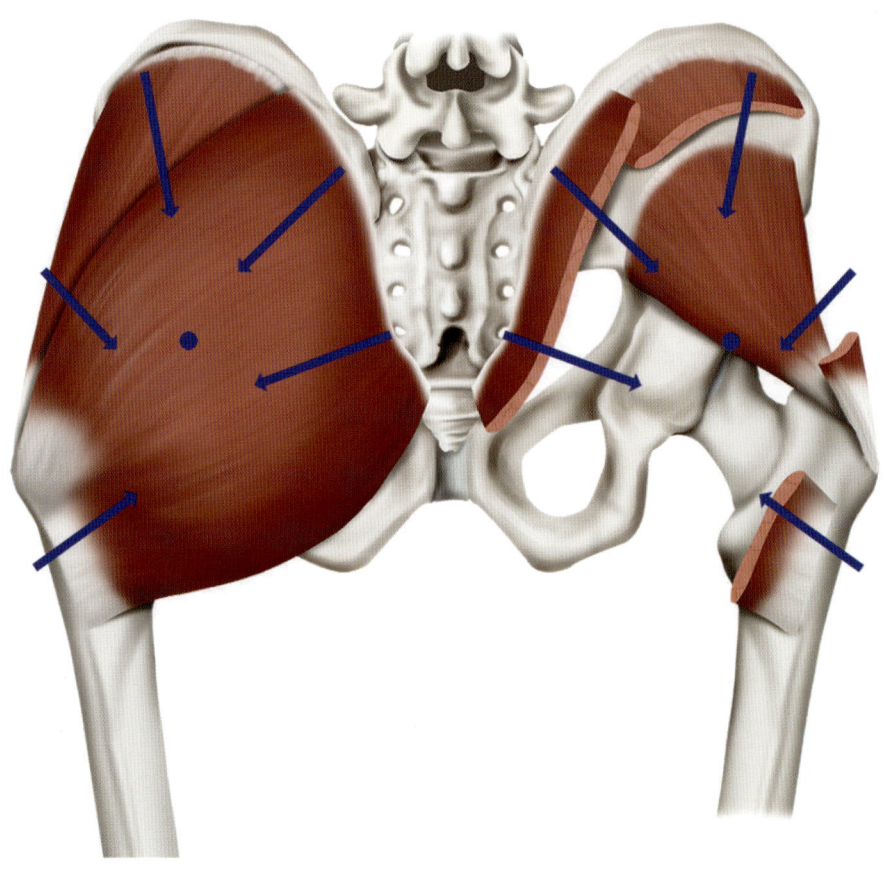

IV. Clinical Cases and Protocols

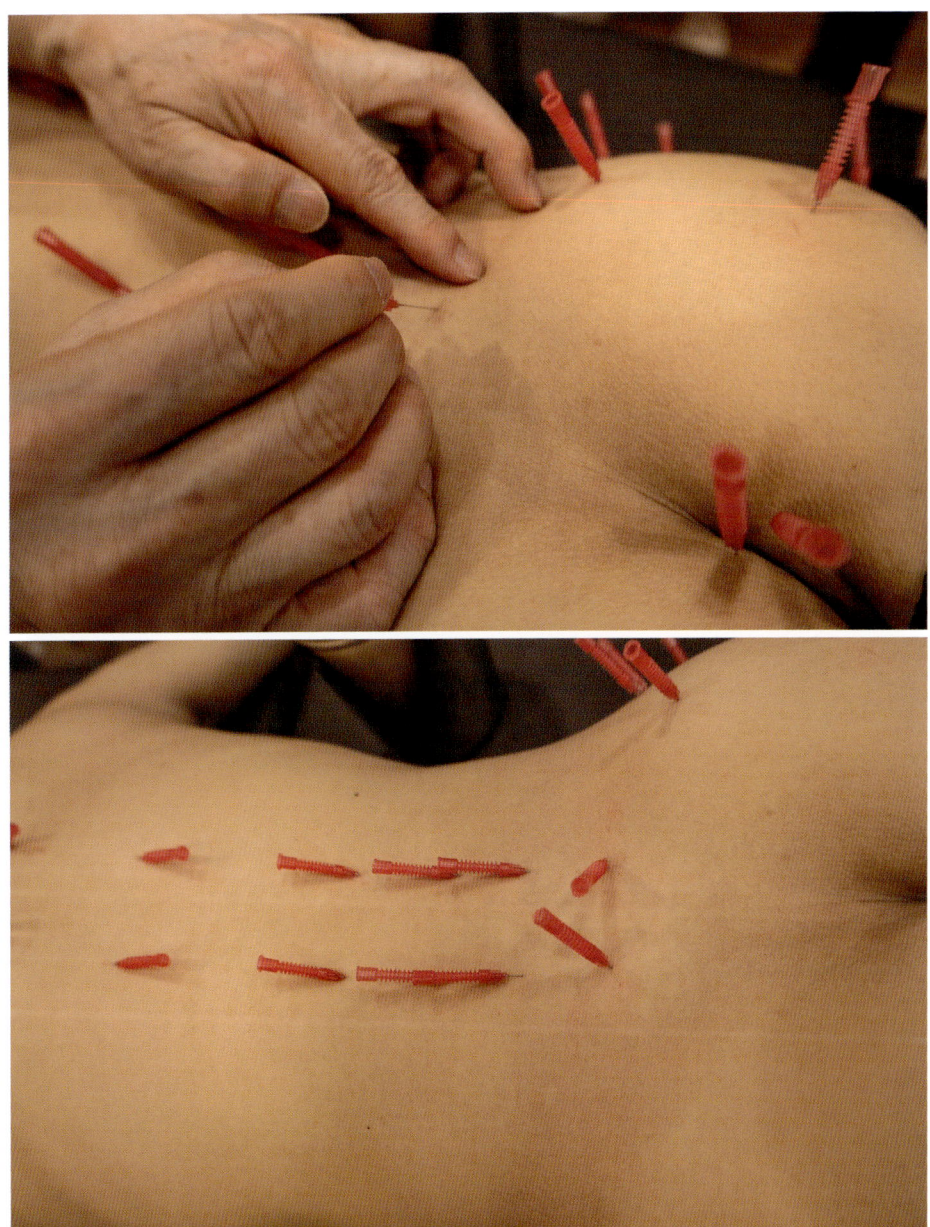

Insert threads obliquely into the sacroiliac joint.

Palpate the posterior superior iliac spine (PSIS), then insert obliquely approximately 1 cm medial to it, in the direction of the iliolumbar ligament.

IV. Clinical Cases and Protocols

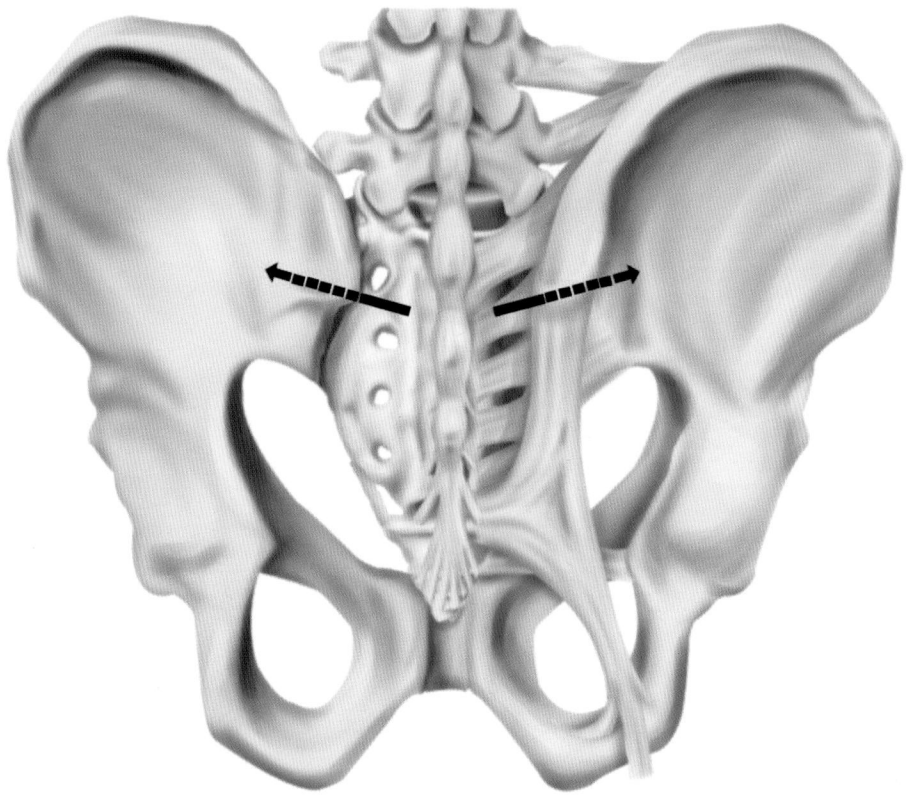

IV. Clinical Cases and Protocols

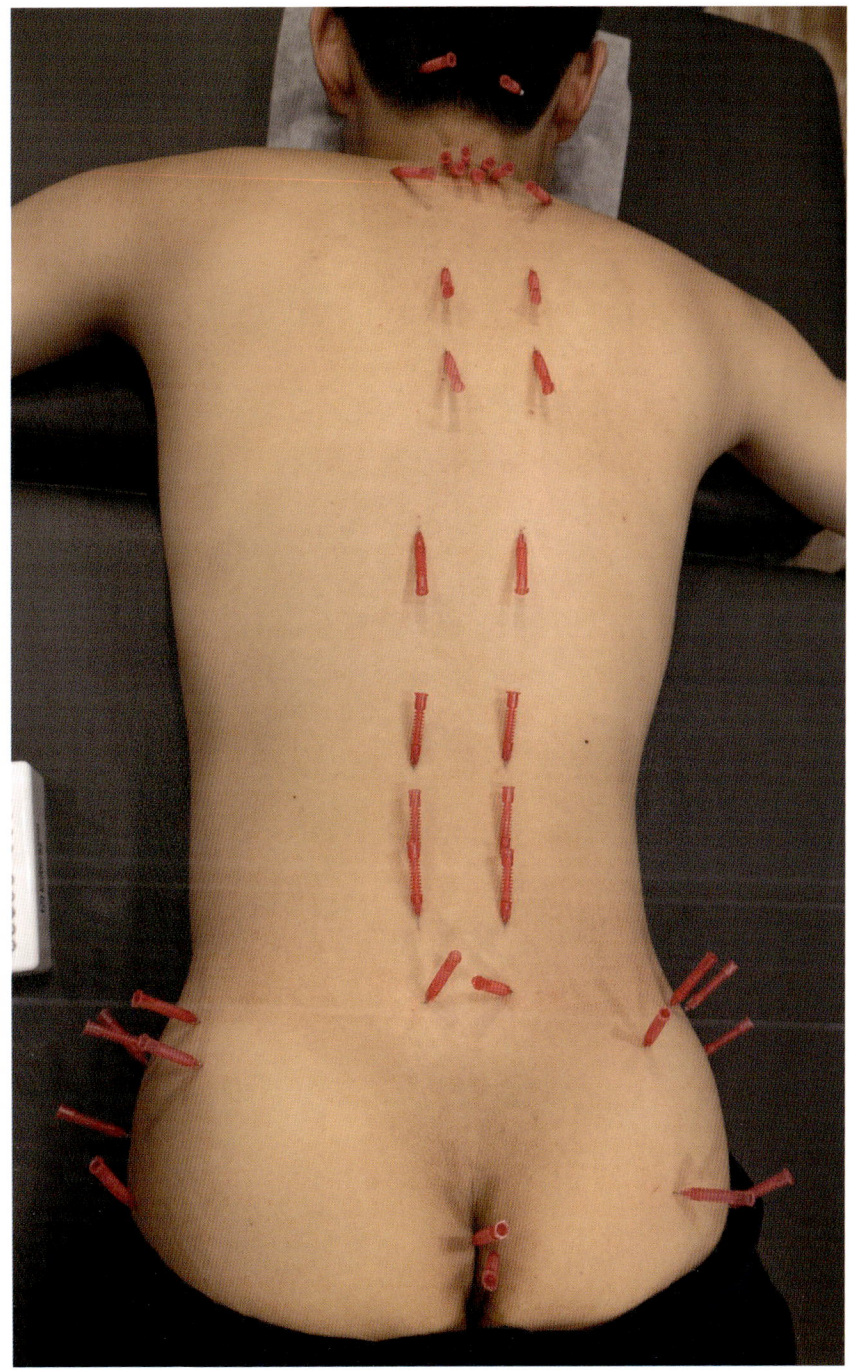

IV. Clinical Cases and Protocols

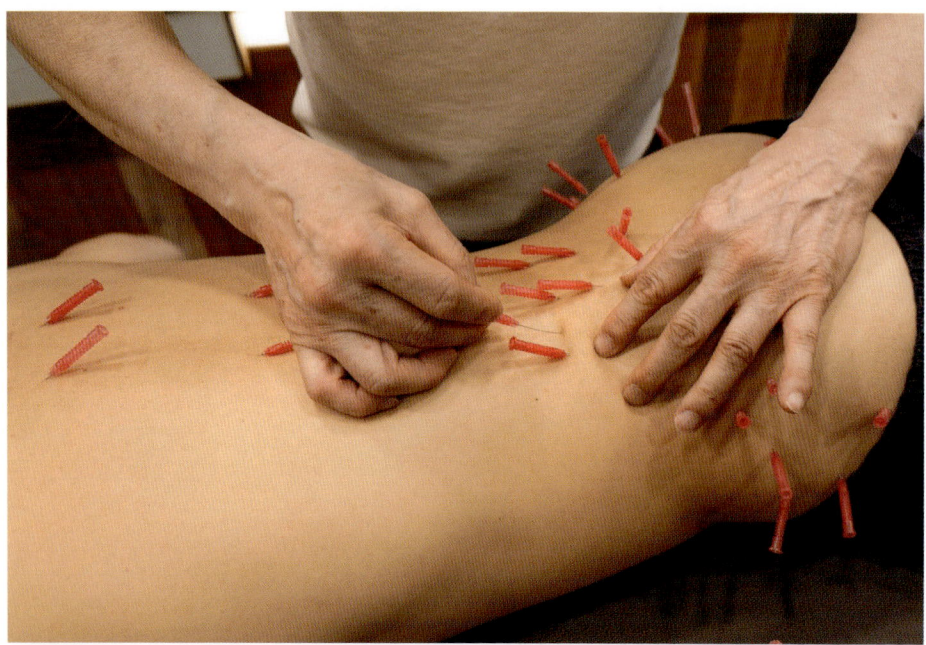

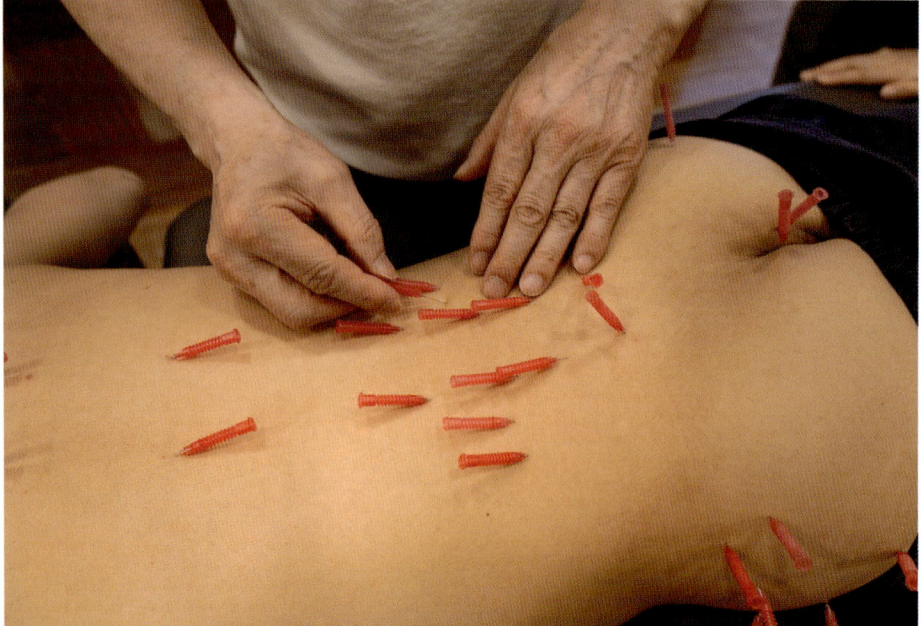

Insert threads transversely targeting the iliocostalis muscle, part of the erector spinae group, which corresponds to Bladder Meridian Line 2.

IV. Clinical Cases and Protocols

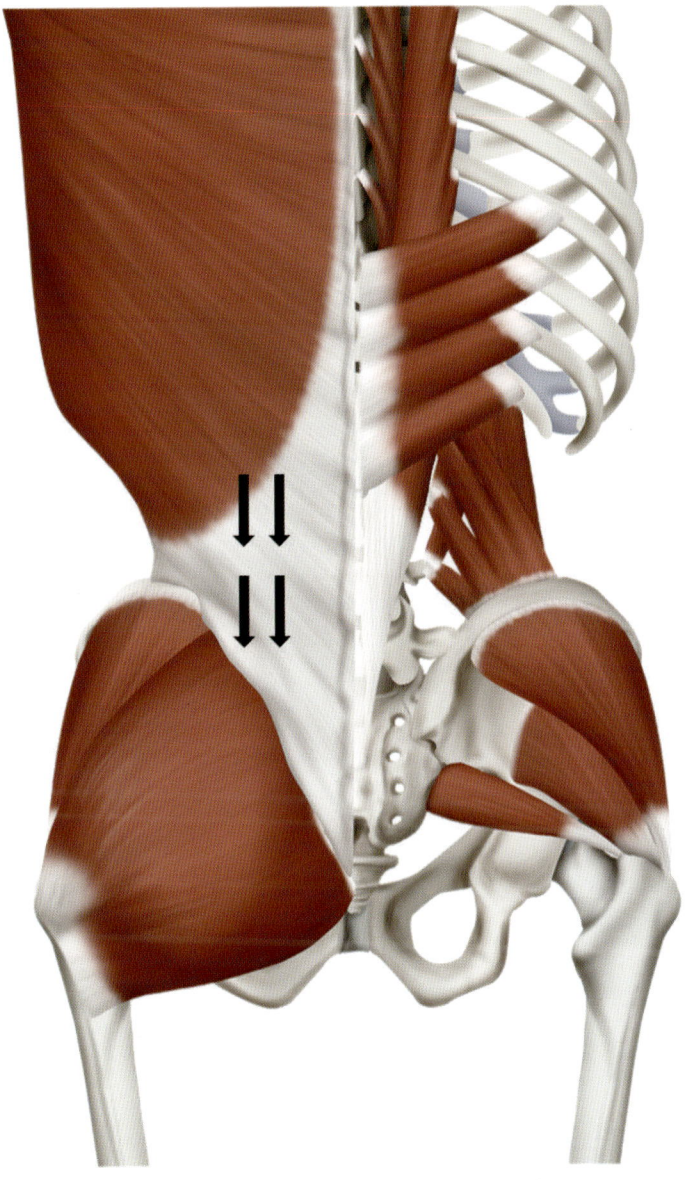

IV. Clinical Cases and Protocols

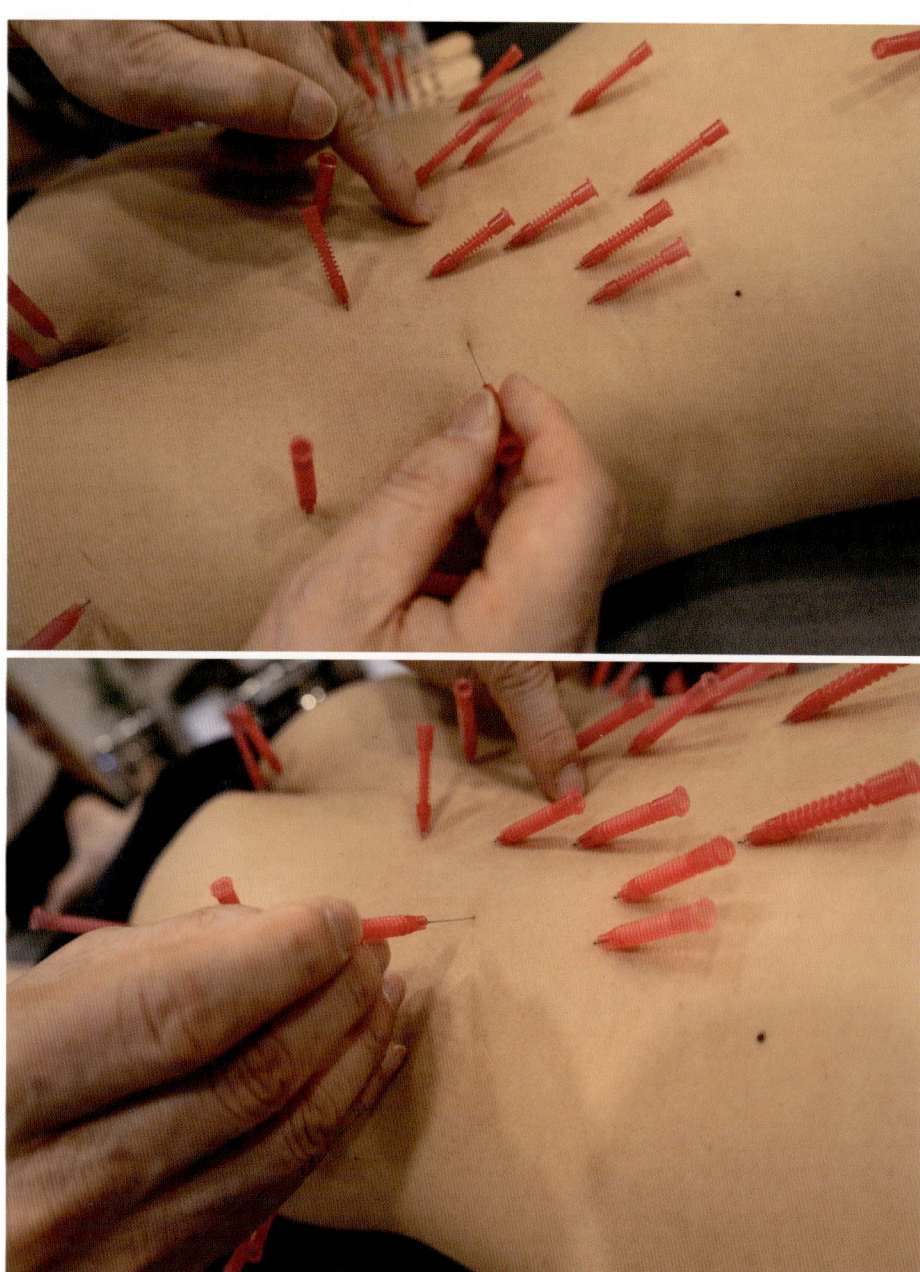

IV. Clinical Cases and Protocols

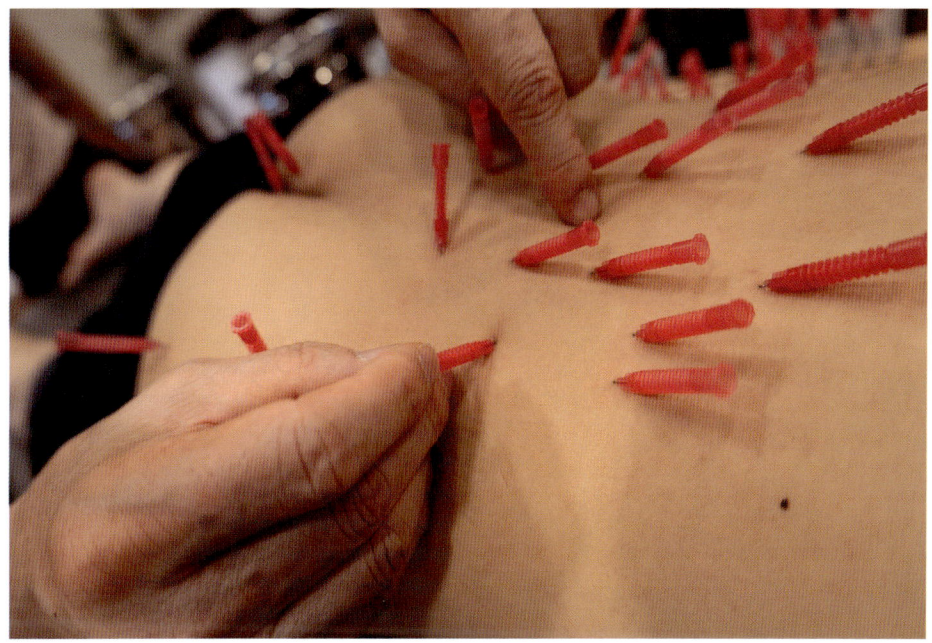

Using a 6 cm thread, insert obliquely from the iliocostalis lumborum toward the vertebral body.
With this approach, it is possible to simultaneously stimulate the iliocostalis lumborum, longissimus, and multifidus muscles in a single insertion.

IV. Clinical Cases and Protocols

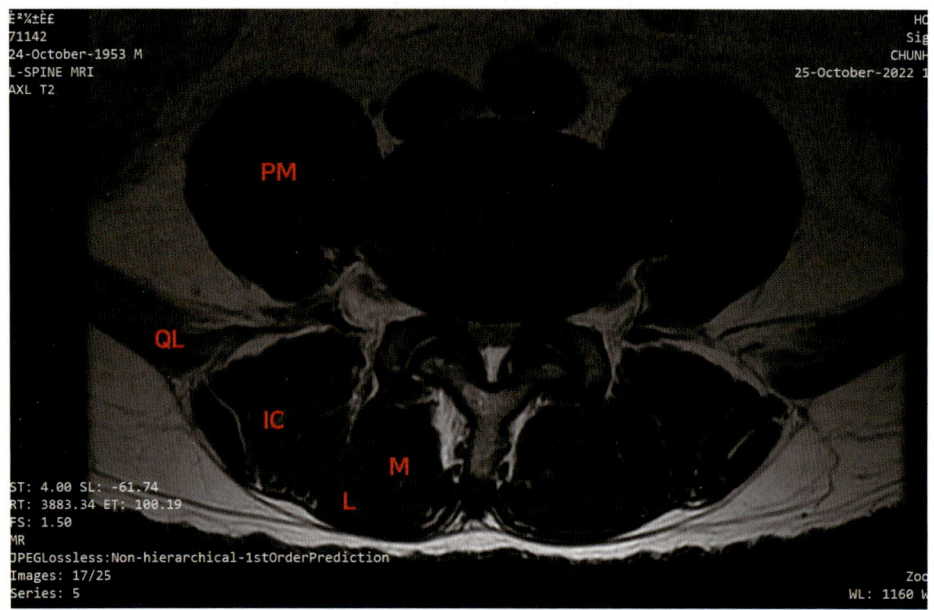

(Quadratus Lumborum MRI)

PM: Psoas Major
M: Multifidus
L: Longissimus Thoracis
IC: Iliocostalis Lumborum
QL: Quadratus Lumborum

IV. Clinical Cases and Protocols

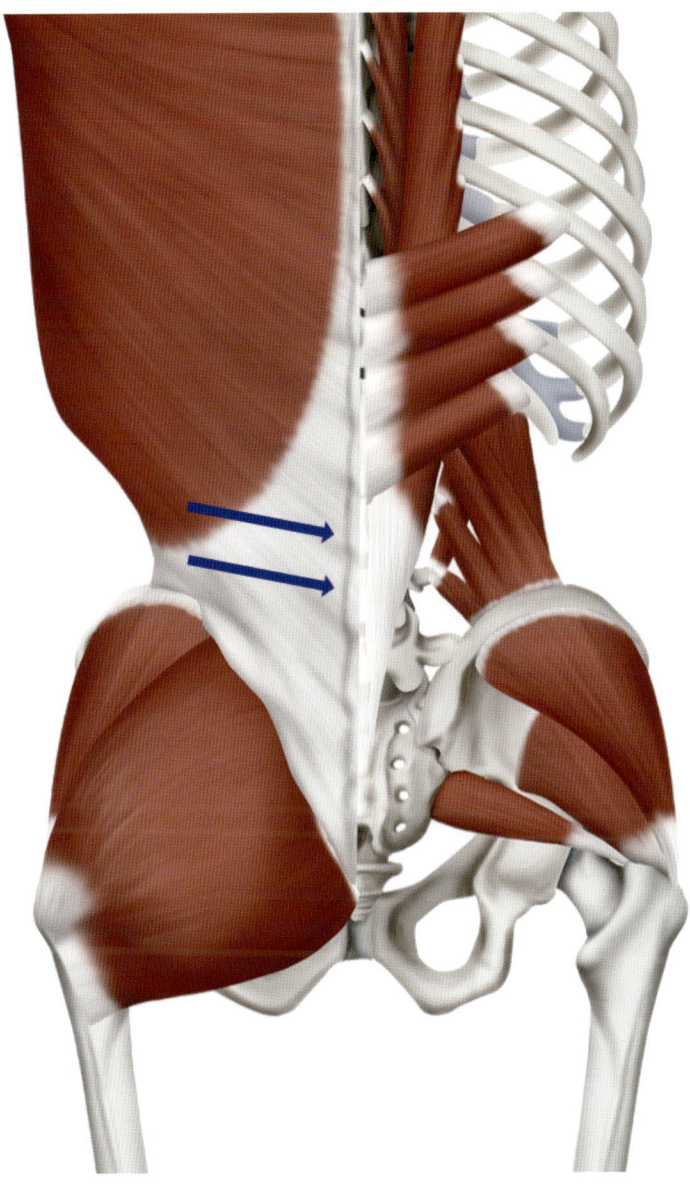

IV. Clinical Cases and Protocols

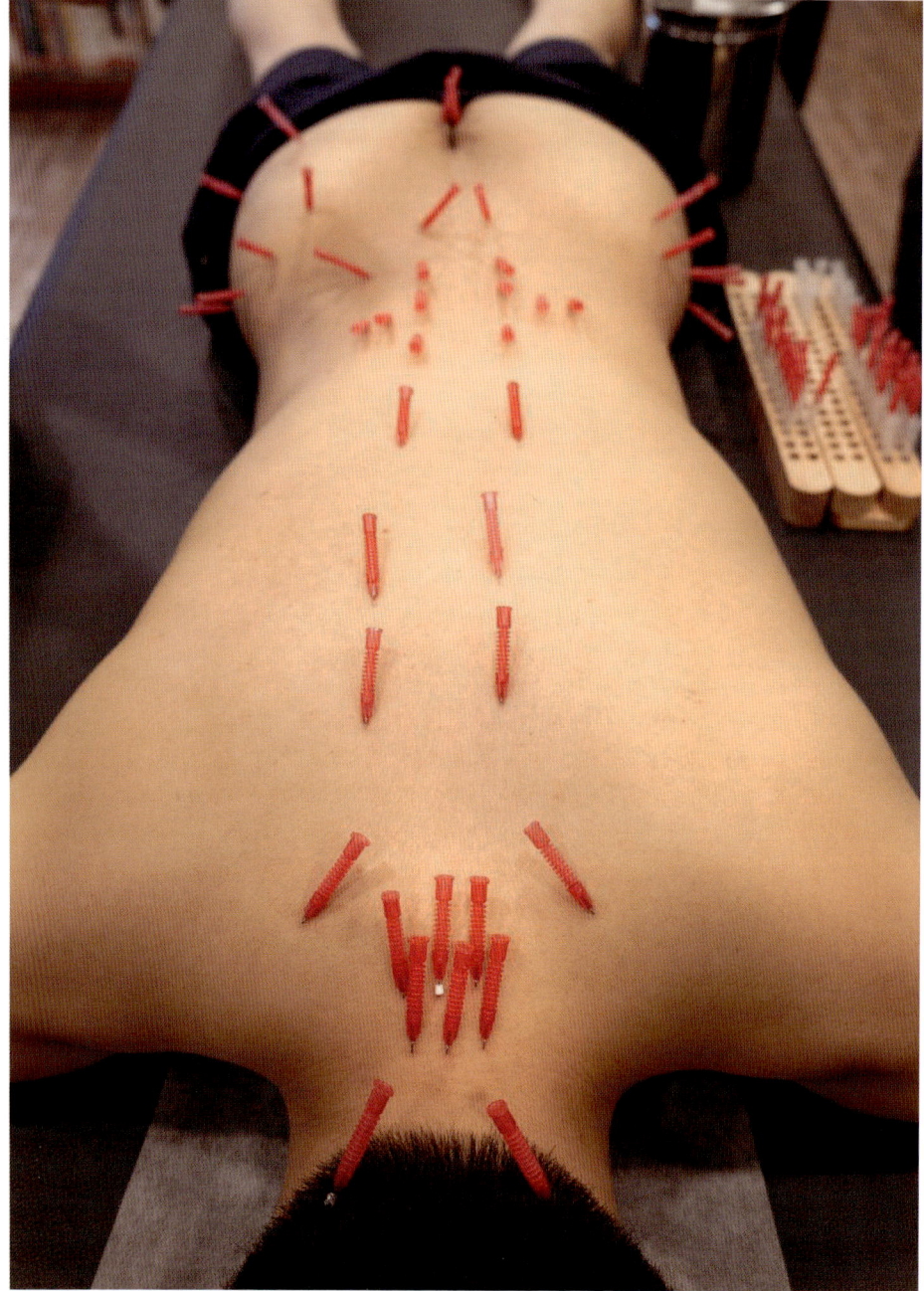

IV. Clinical Cases and Protocols

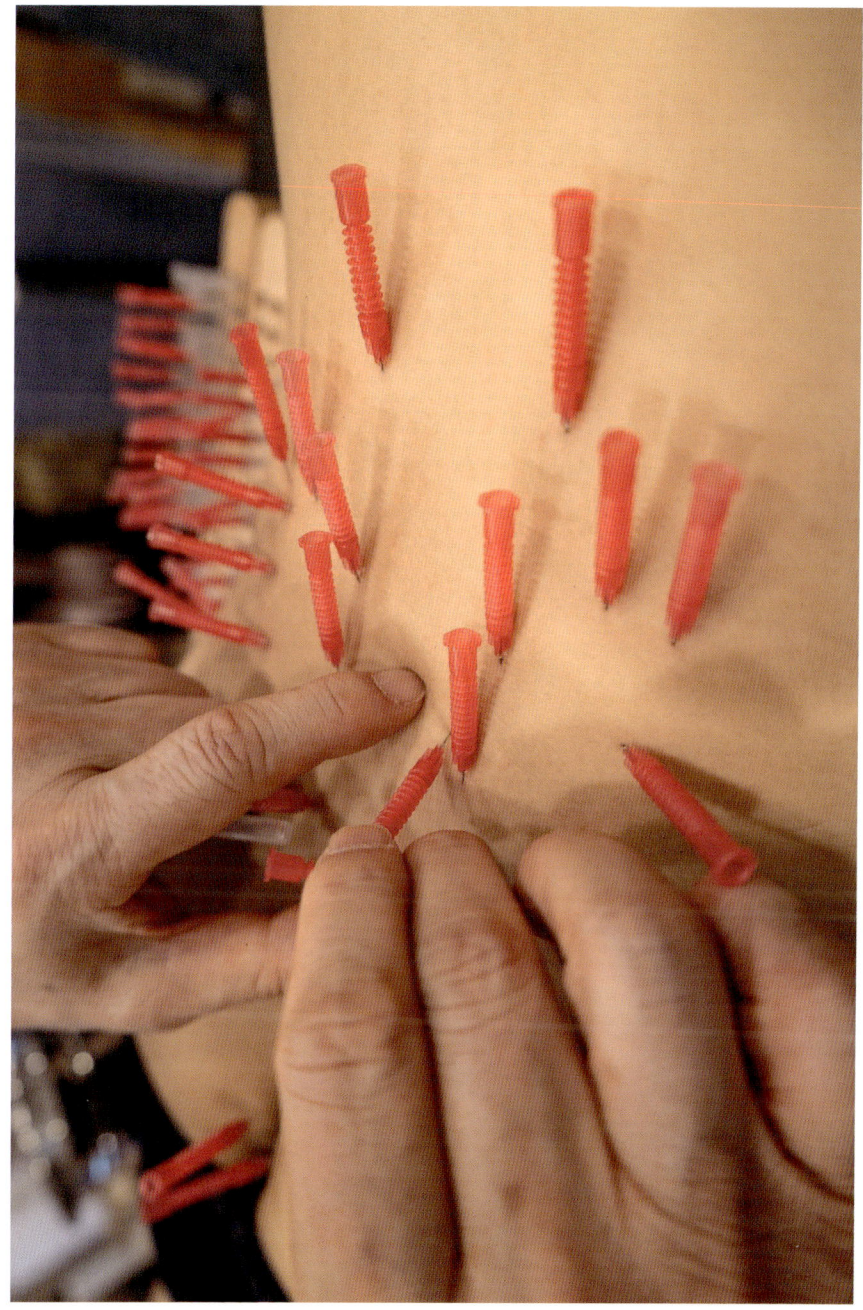

IV. Clinical Cases and Protocols

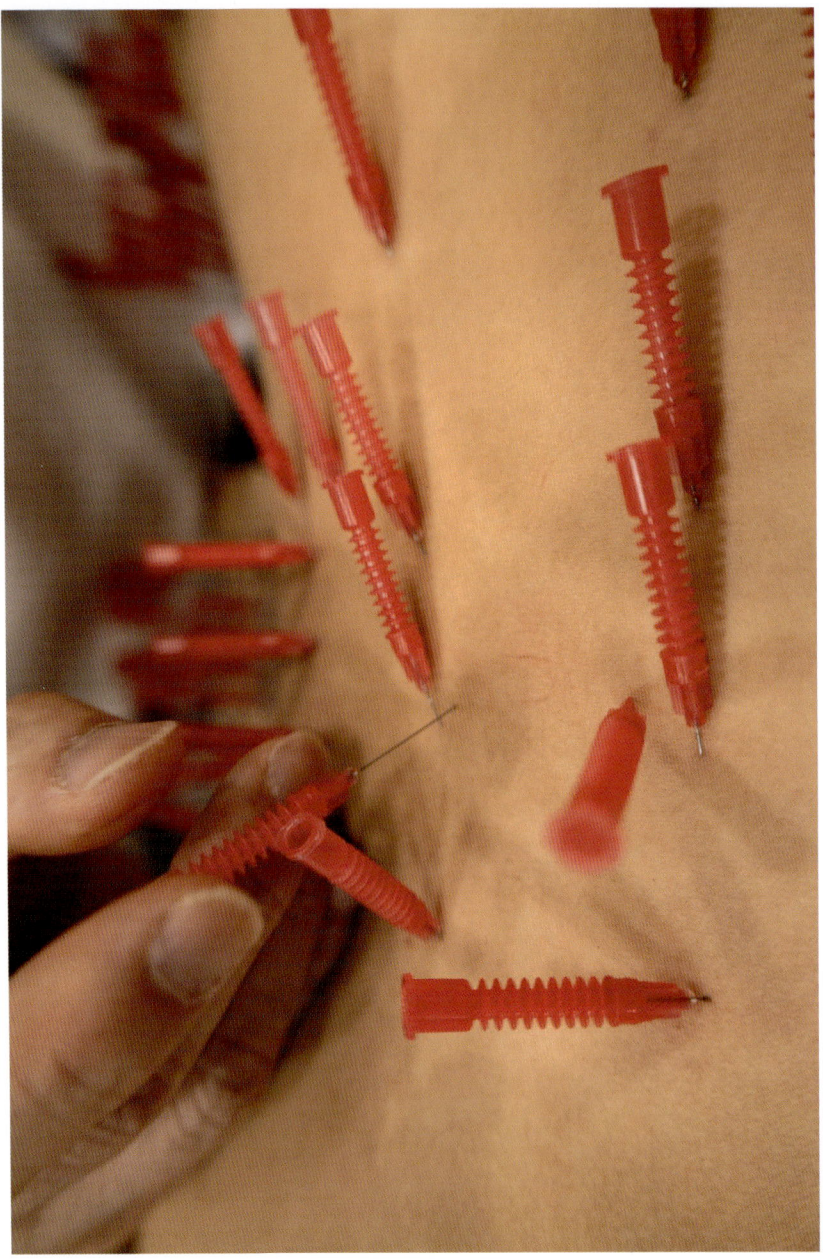

Insert perpendicularly toward the vertebral body, targeting the multifidus muscle approximately 1 cm lateral to the spinous process of the lumbar vertebra—corresponding to the Huatuojiaji points.

IV. Clinical Cases and Protocols

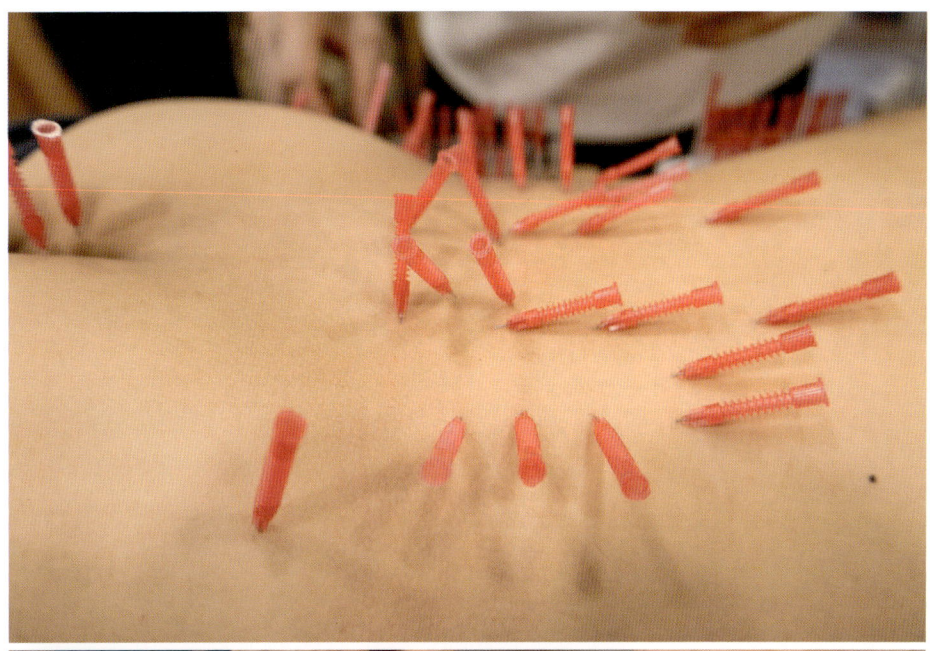

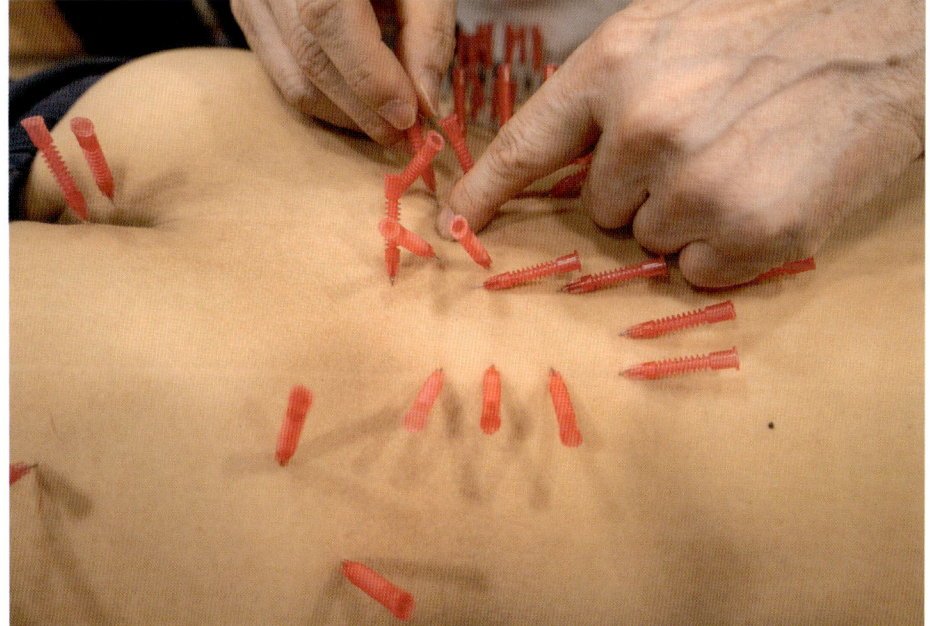

IV. Clinical Cases and Protocols

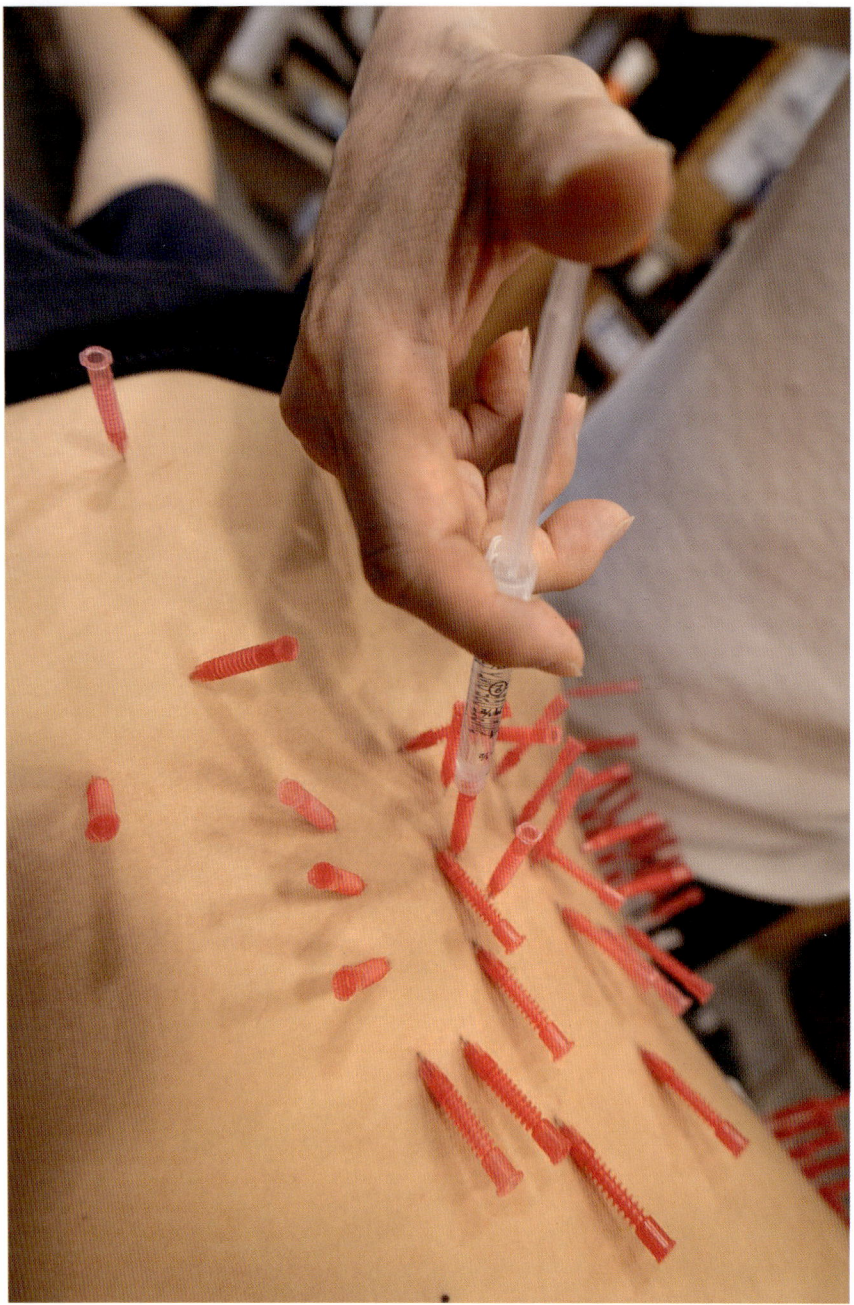

IV. Clinical Cases and Protocols

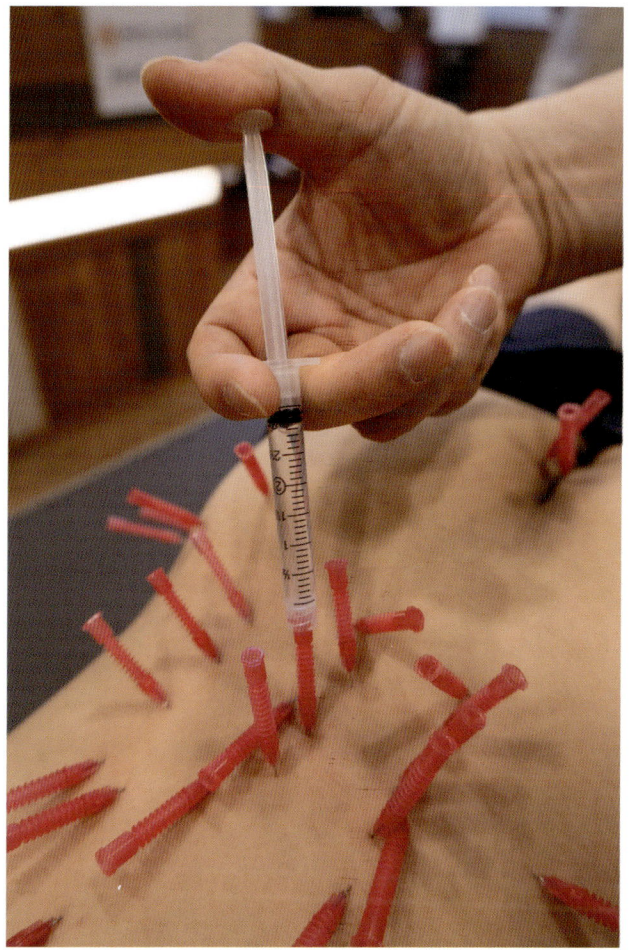

Inject 3cc of pharmacopuncture into each site where the threads have been inserted perpendicularly into the multifidus muscles.

When thread embedding is combined with pharmacopuncture, the following synergistic effects can be expected:

· Pain relief and anti-inflammatory effects: The anti-inflammatory and analgesic properties of pharmacopuncture help reduce discomfort and inflammatory responses at the thread insertion sites.

· Tissue regeneration and improved circulation: Pharmacopuncture promotes tissue repair and enhances blood flow, creating a more favorable environment for the degradation and absorption of the threads within the body.

IV. Clinical Cases and Protocols

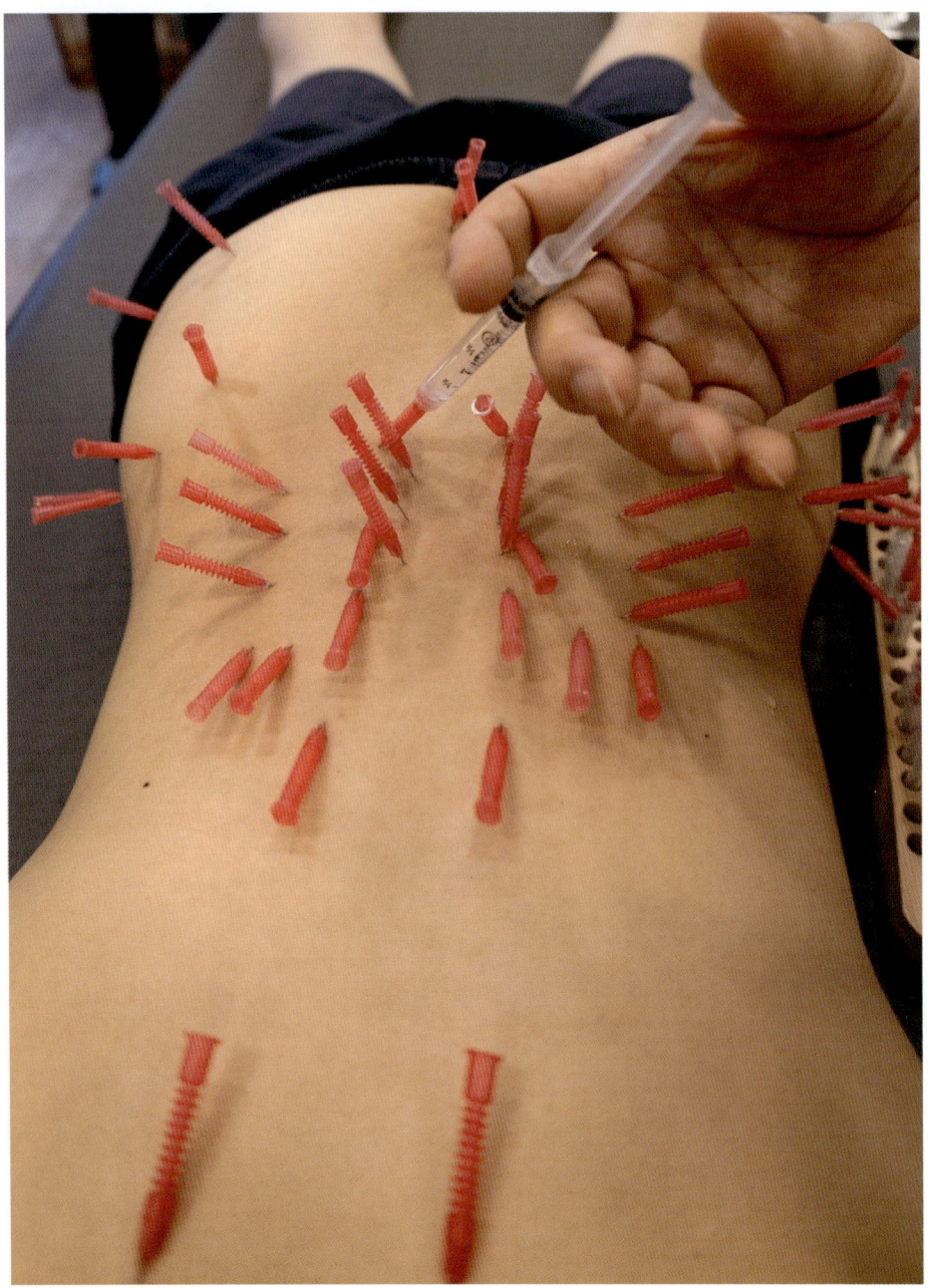

Perform thread embedding and pharmacopuncture simultaneously at the sacroiliac joint.

IV. Clinical Cases and Protocols

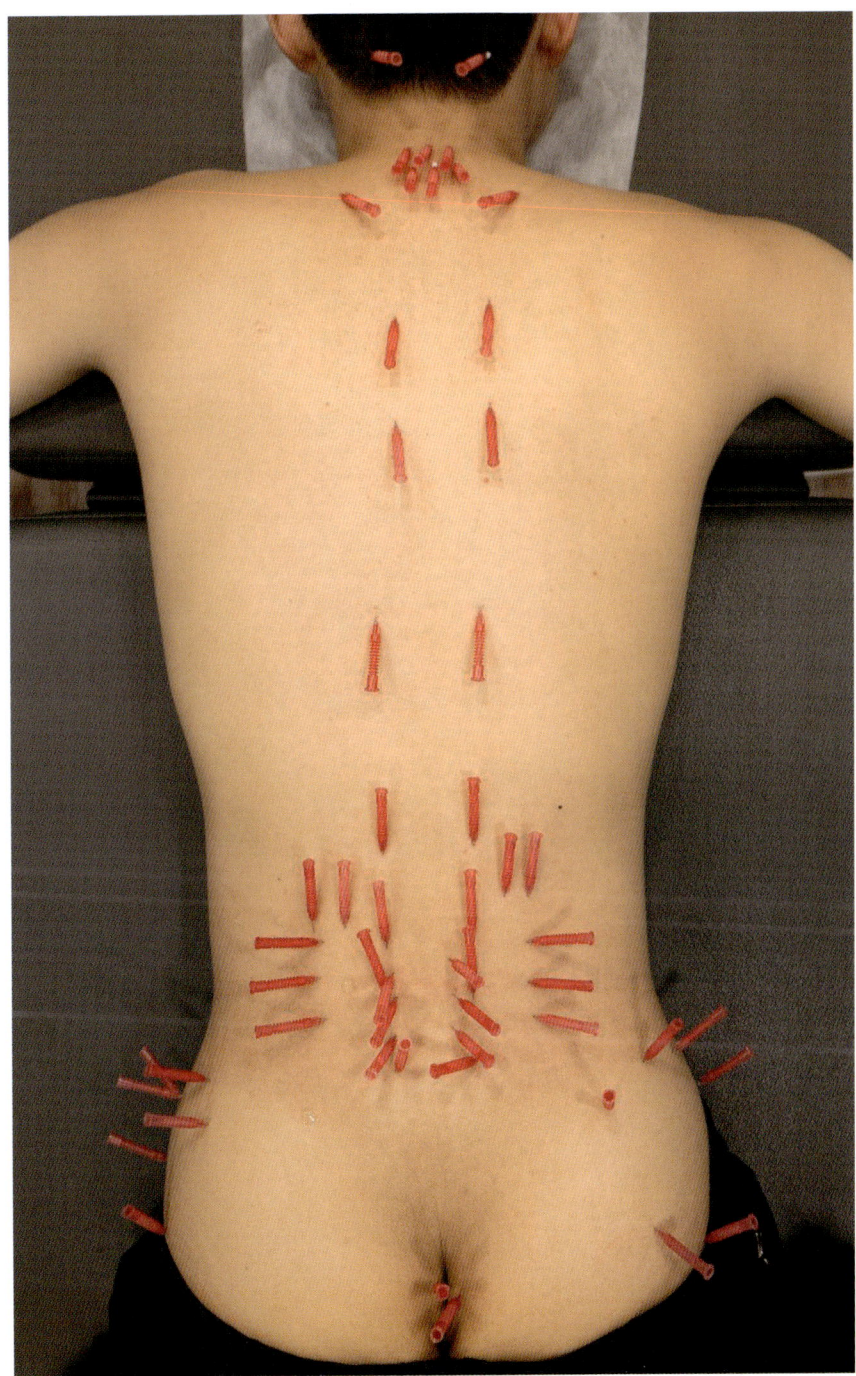

IV. Clinical Cases and Protocols

2. Pelvic Region

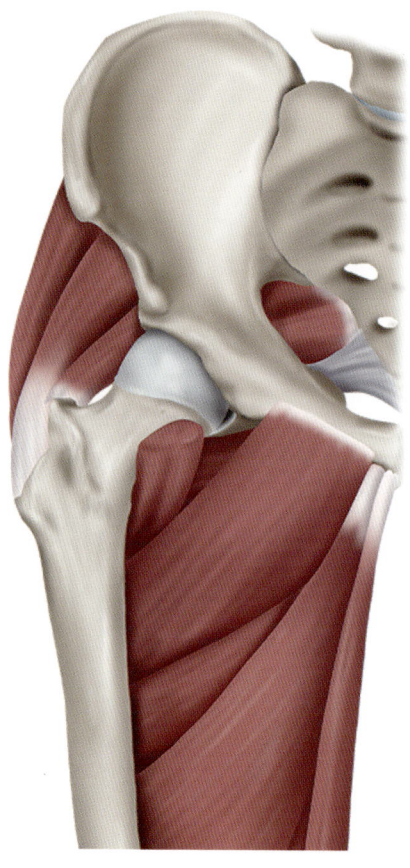
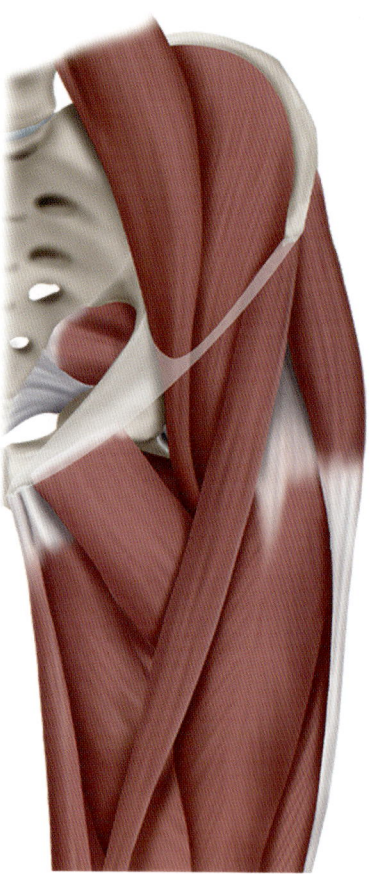

IV. Clinical Cases and Protocols

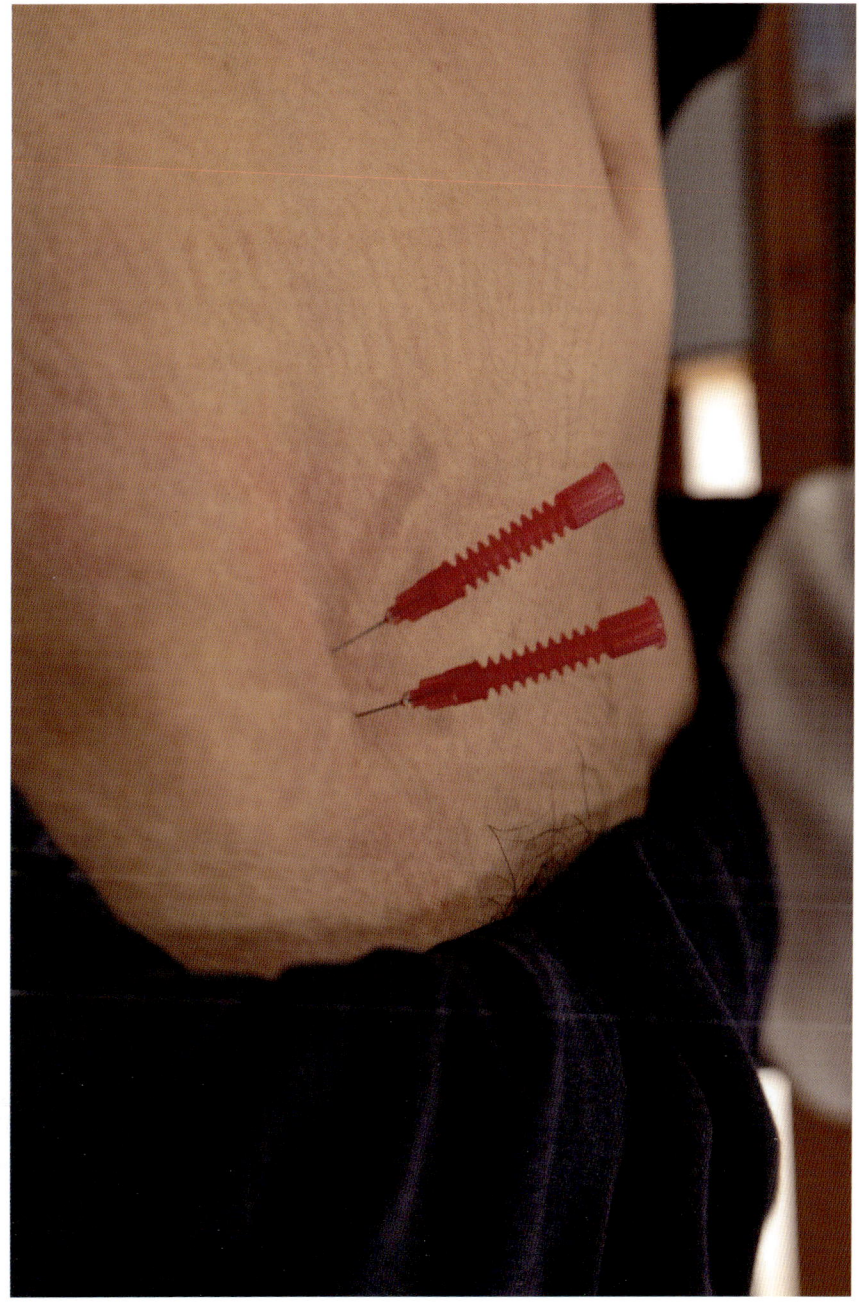

IV. Clinical Cases and Protocols

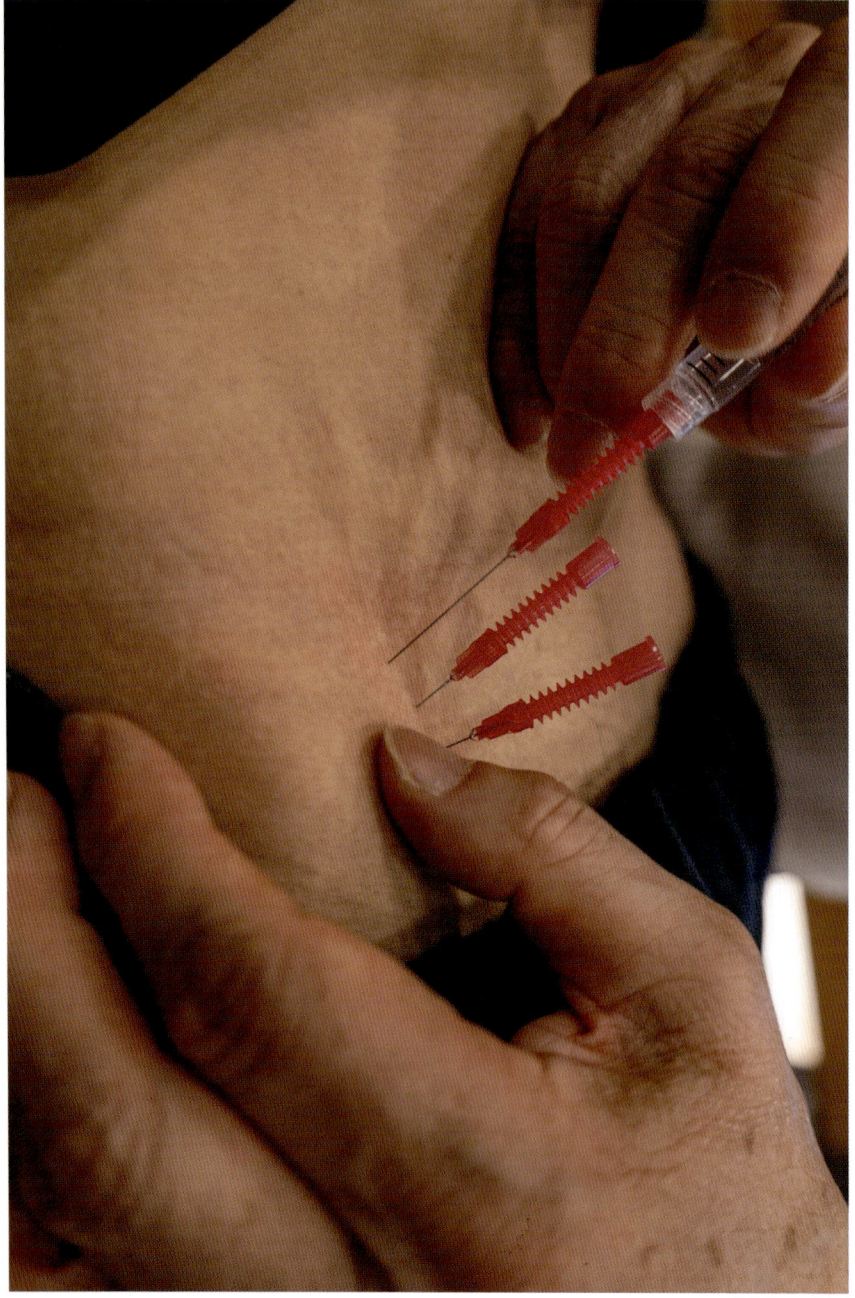

IV. Clinical Cases and Protocols

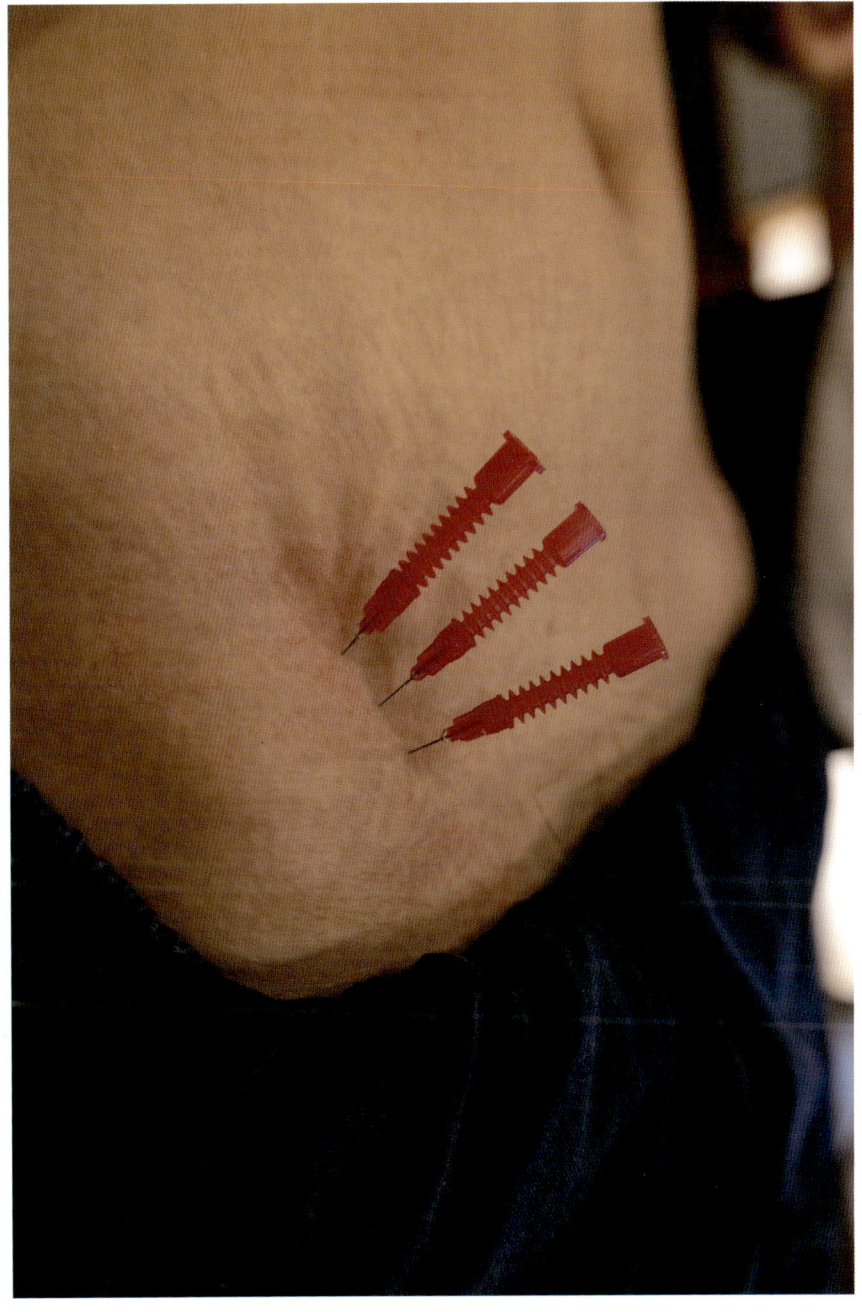

IV. Clinical Cases and Protocols

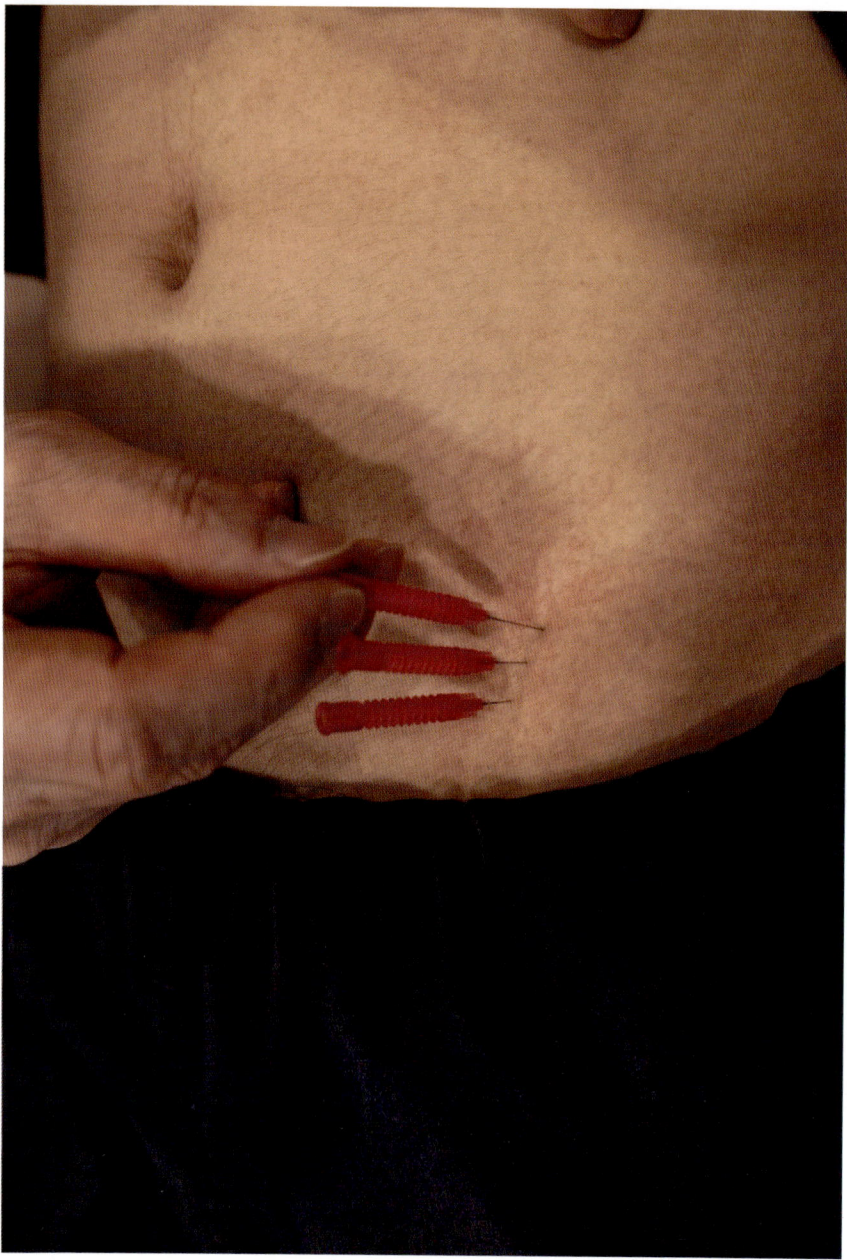

Palpate the anterior superior iliac spine (ASIS) and insert the thread and 3cc of pharmacopuncture simultaneously along the inner surface of the bone, targeting the iliacus muscle, a part of the iliopsoas group.

IV. Clinical Cases and Protocols

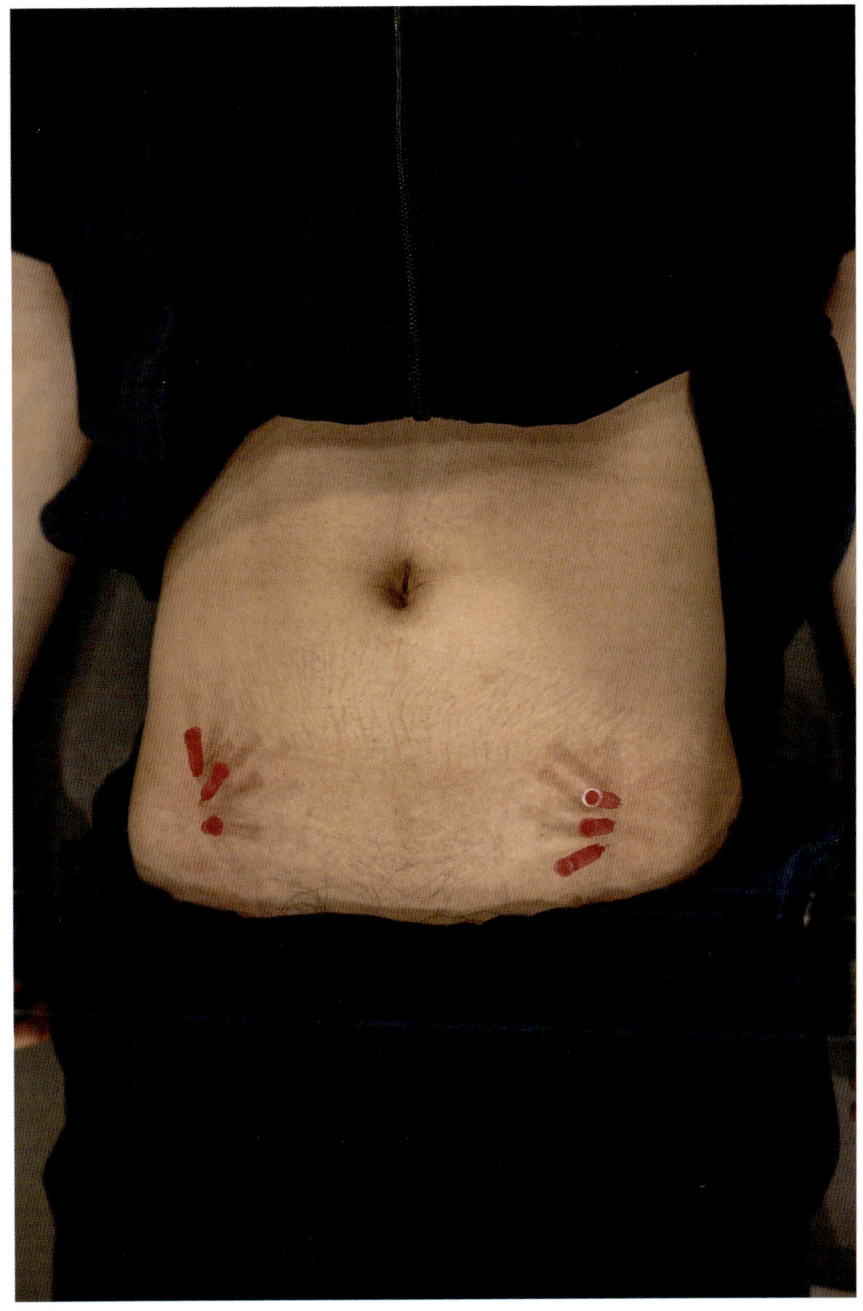

IV. Clinical Cases and Protocols

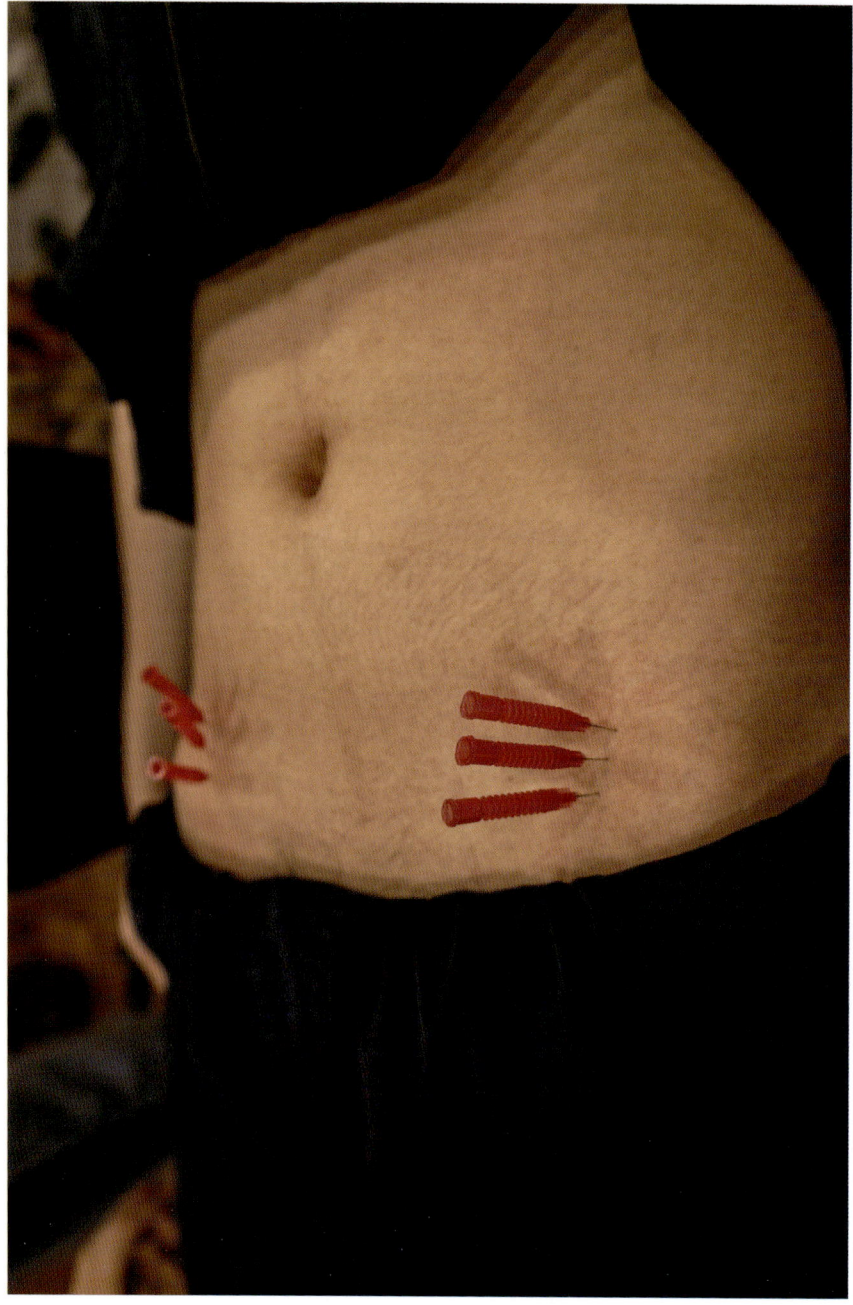

IV. Clinical Cases and Protocols

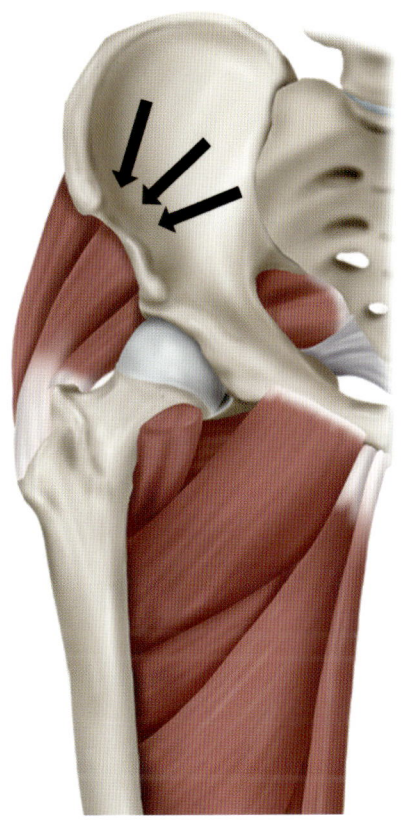
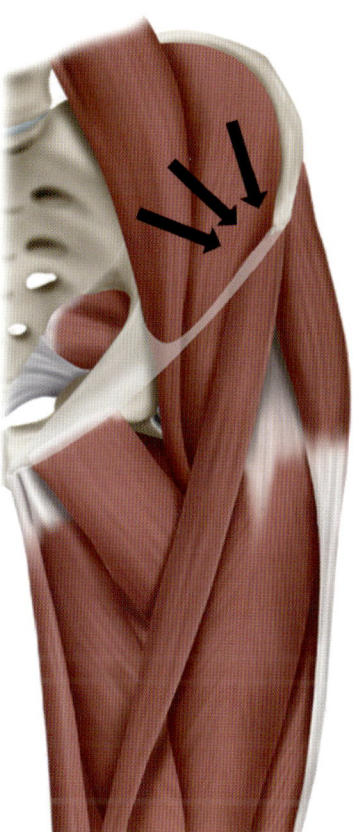

IV. Clinical Cases and Protocols

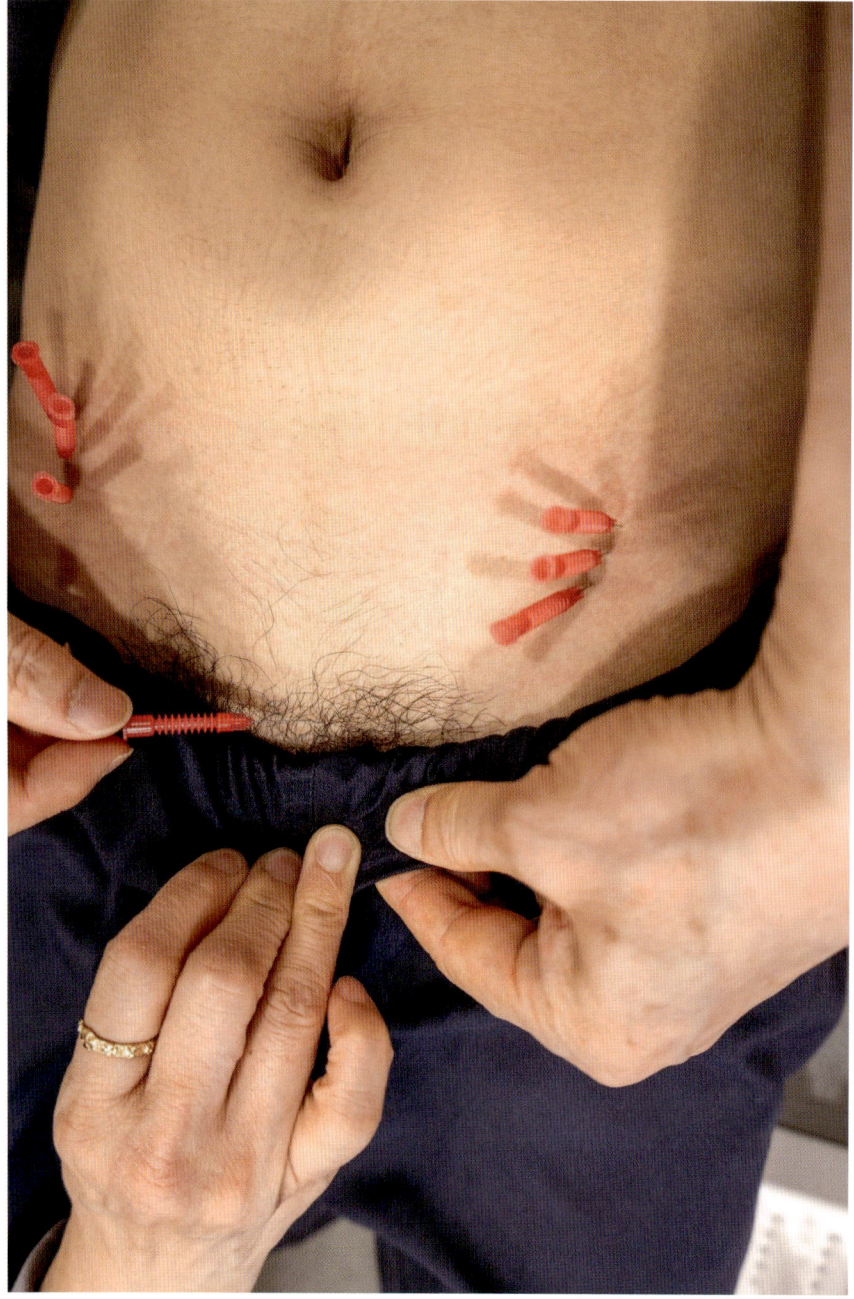

IV. Clinical Cases and Protocols

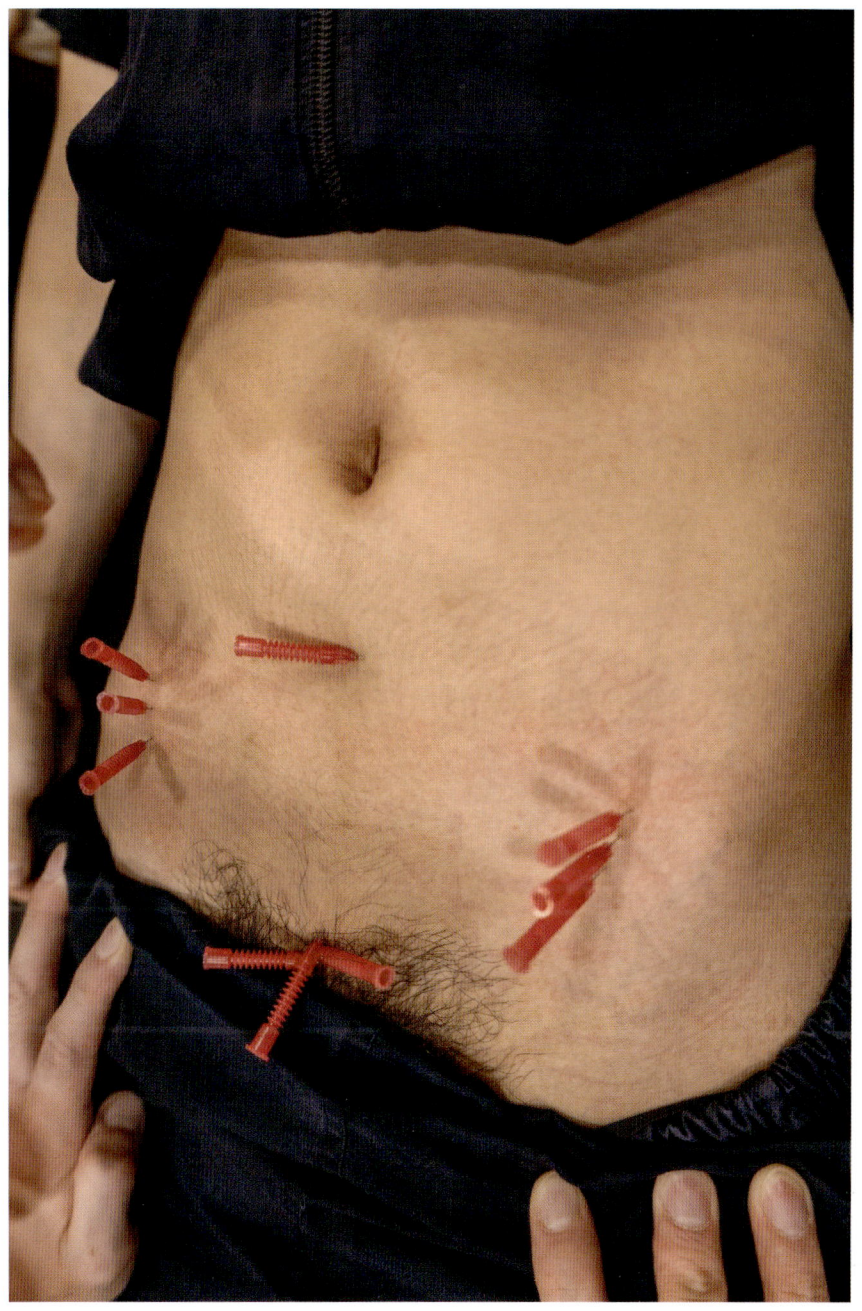

IV. Clinical Cases and Protocols

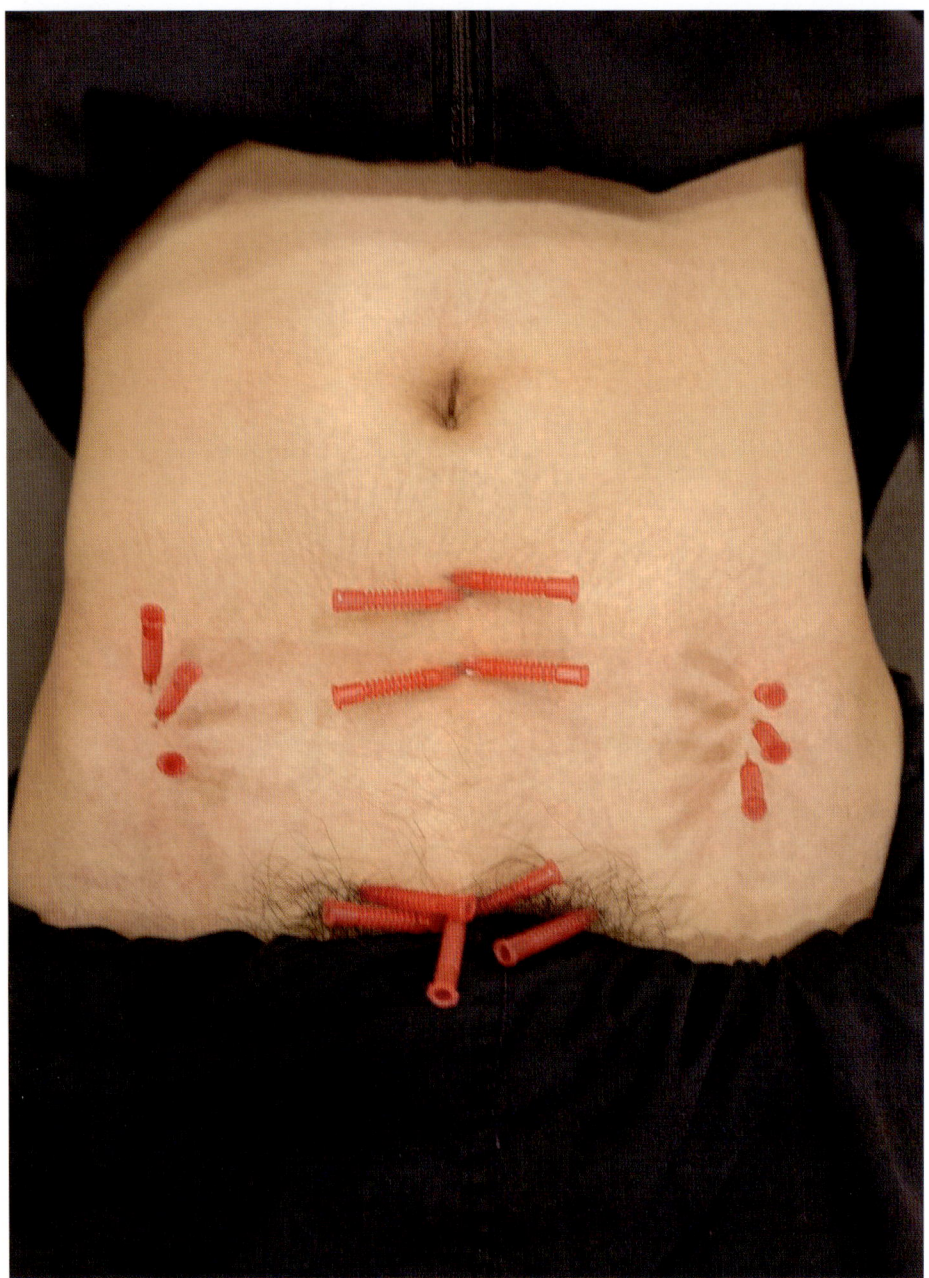

Insert threads transversely into the transverse abdominis fascia, rectus abdominis fascia, and linea alba along the superior border of the pubic region.

IV. Clinical Cases and Protocols

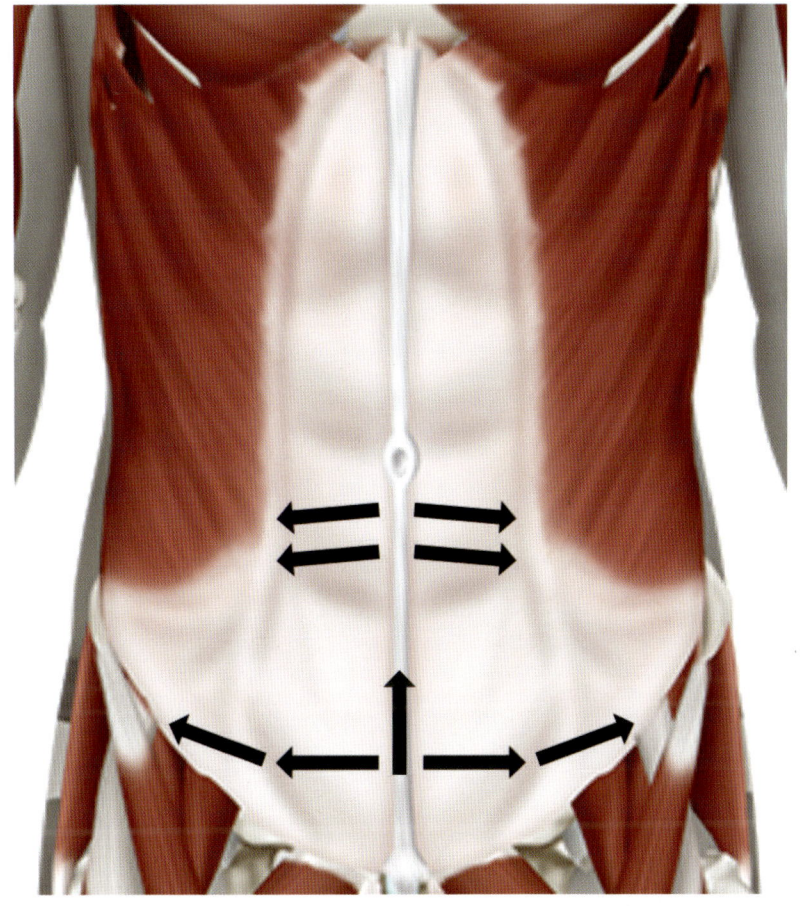

IV. Clinical Cases and Protocols

3. Knee Joint

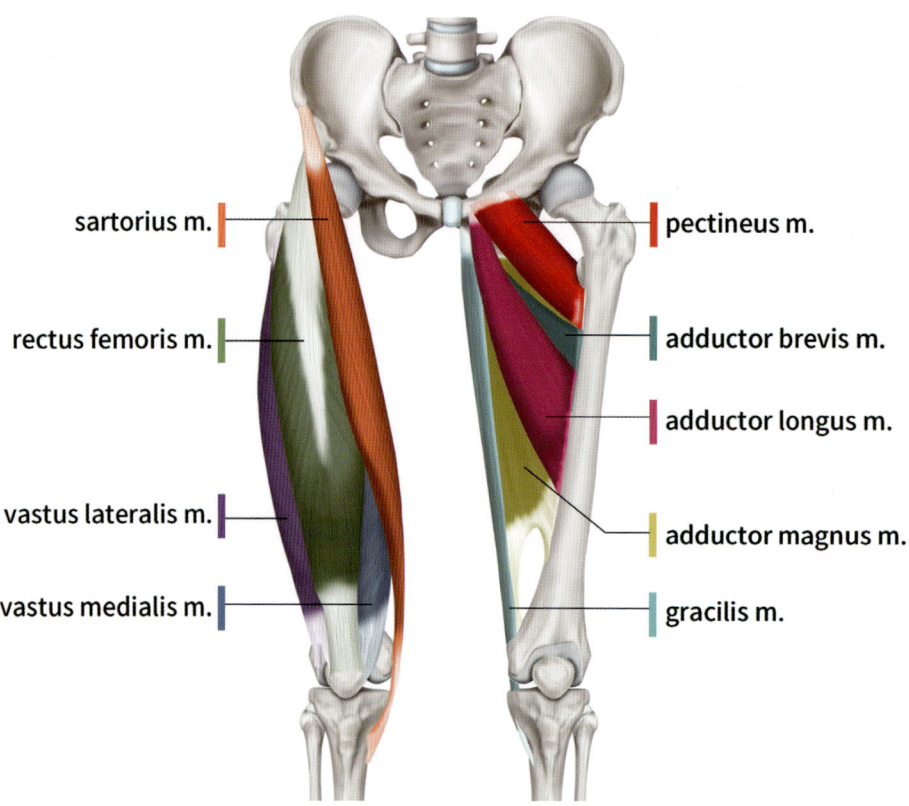

IV. Clinical Cases and Protocols

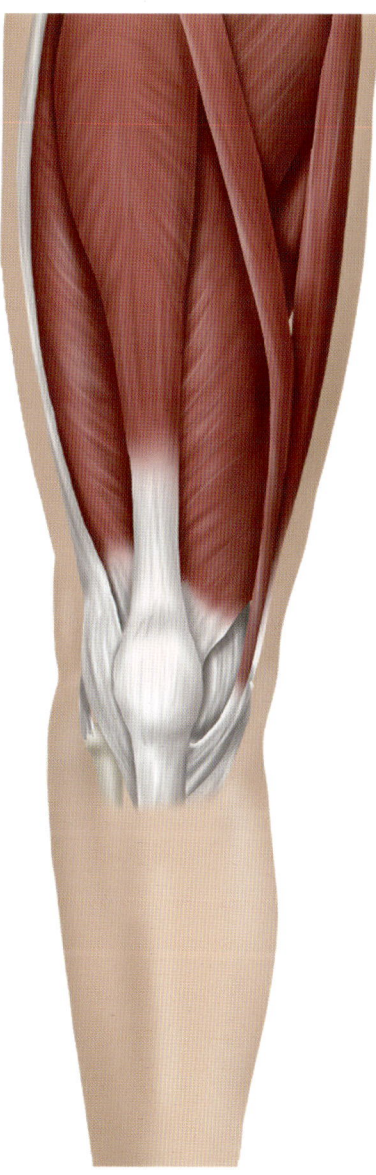

IV. Clinical Cases and Protocols

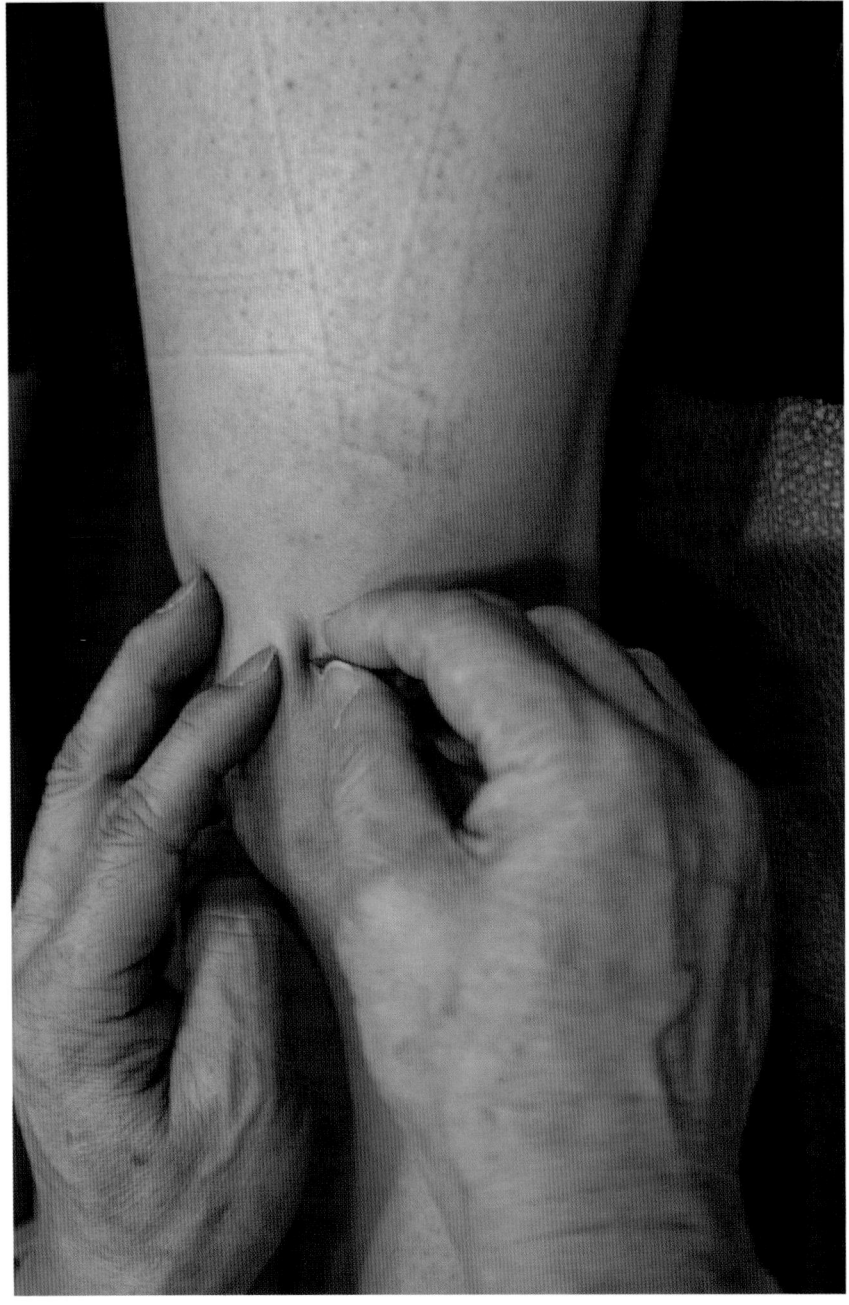

IV. Clinical Cases and Protocols

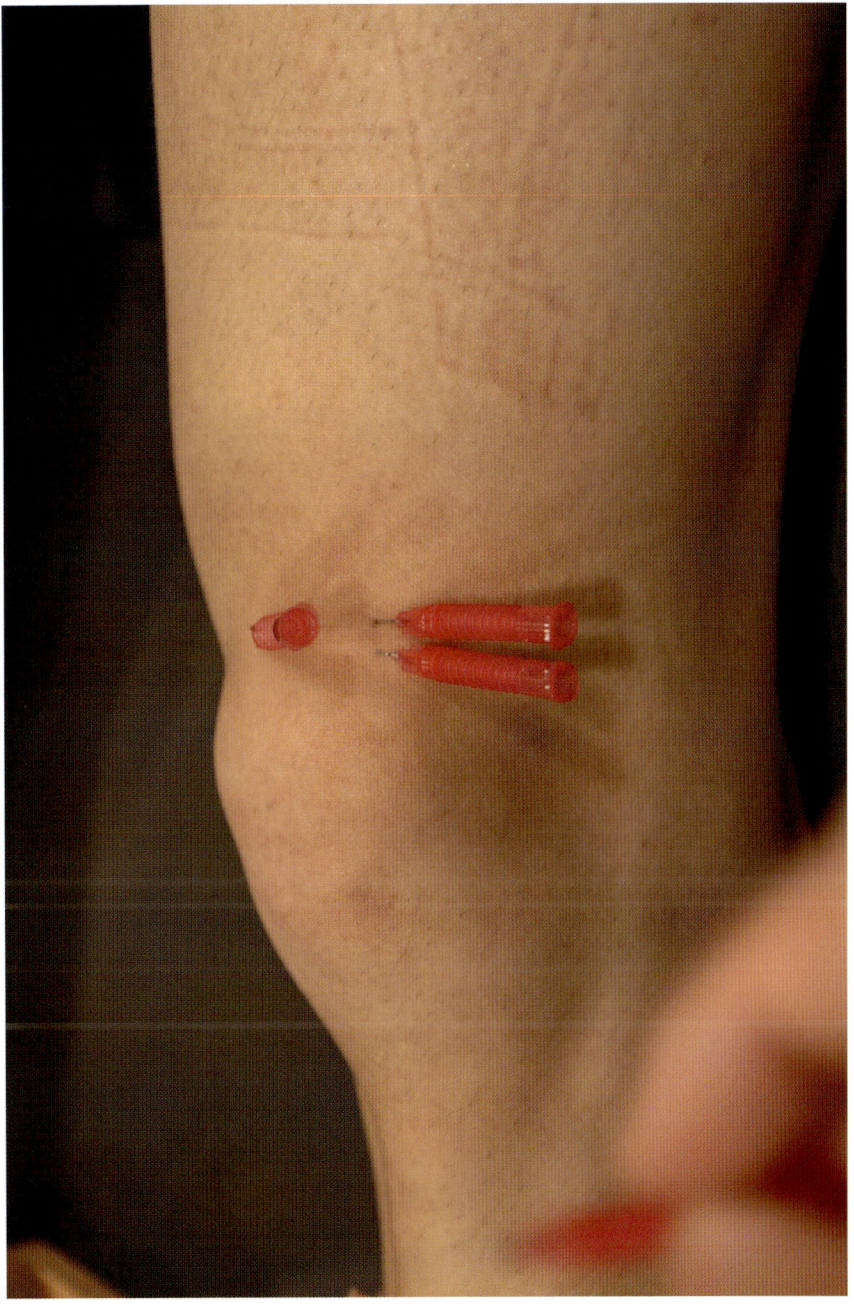

IV. Clinical Cases and Protocols

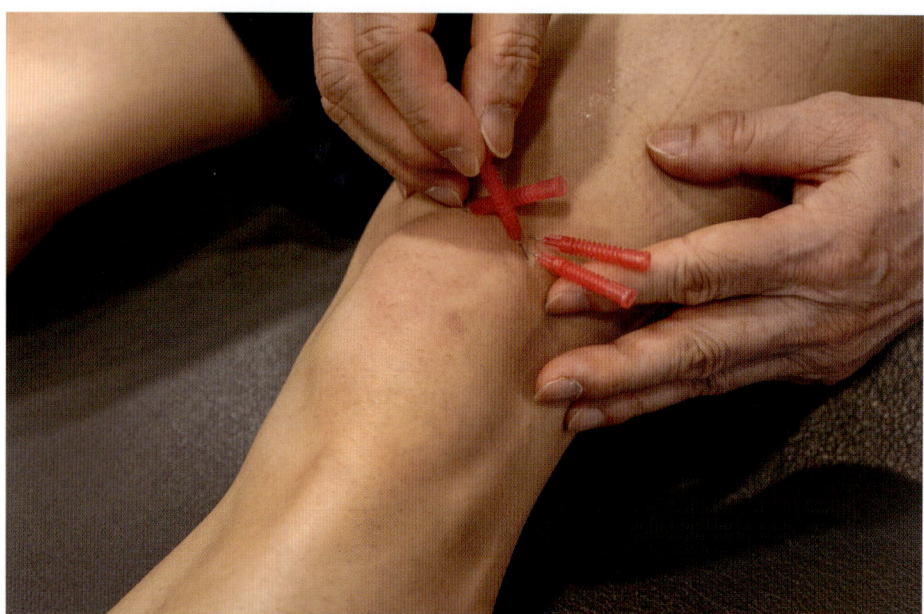

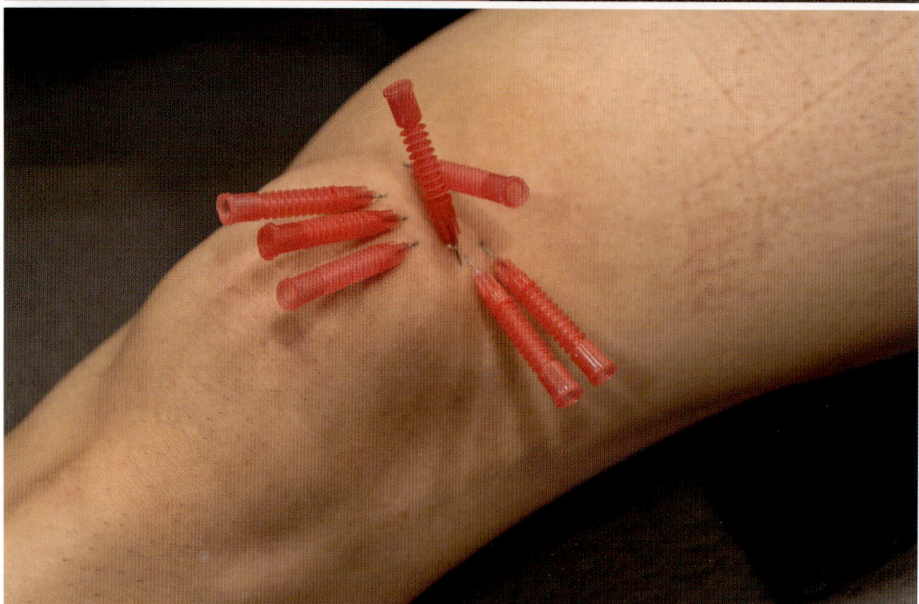

Insert threads transversely over the quadriceps femoris tendon above the patella, and continue transverse insertions toward the vastus medialis and vastus lateralis.
Then, perform a crosshatch pattern of thread embedding toward the origin of the rectus femoris.

IV. Clinical Cases and Protocols

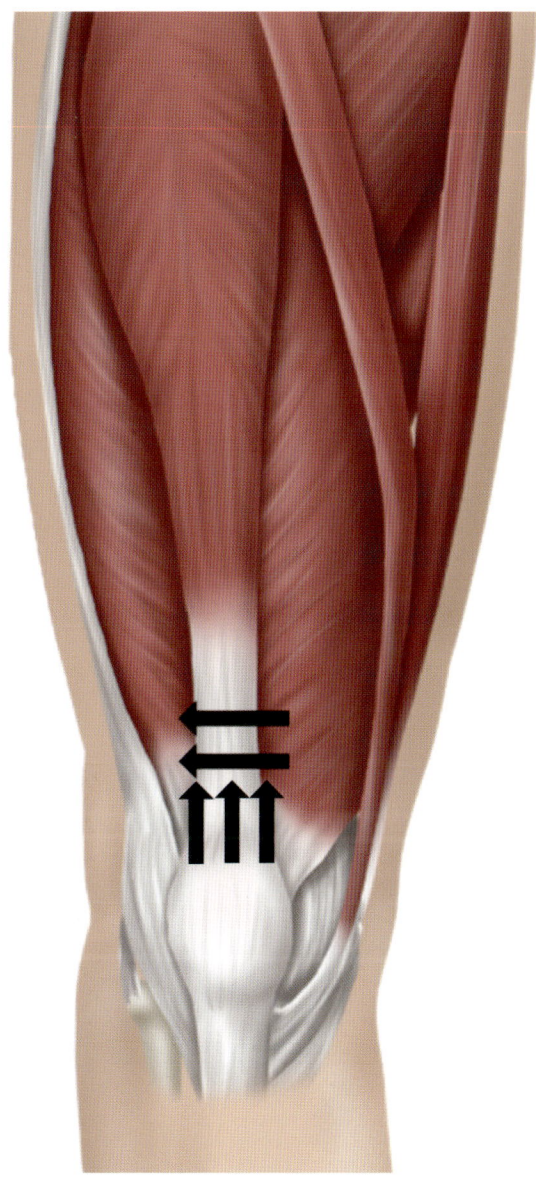

IV. Clinical Cases and Protocols

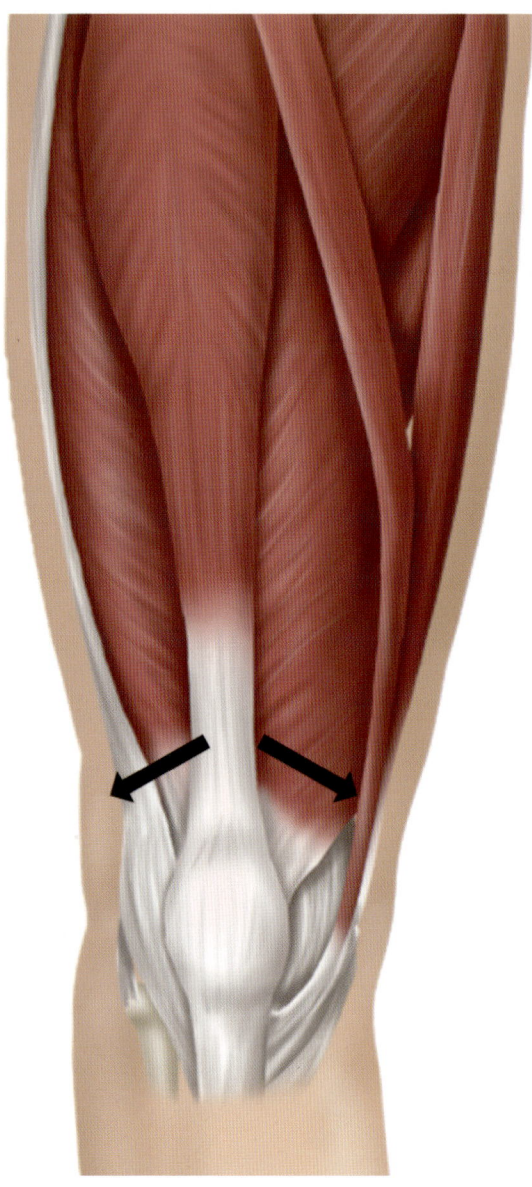

IV. Clinical Cases and Protocols

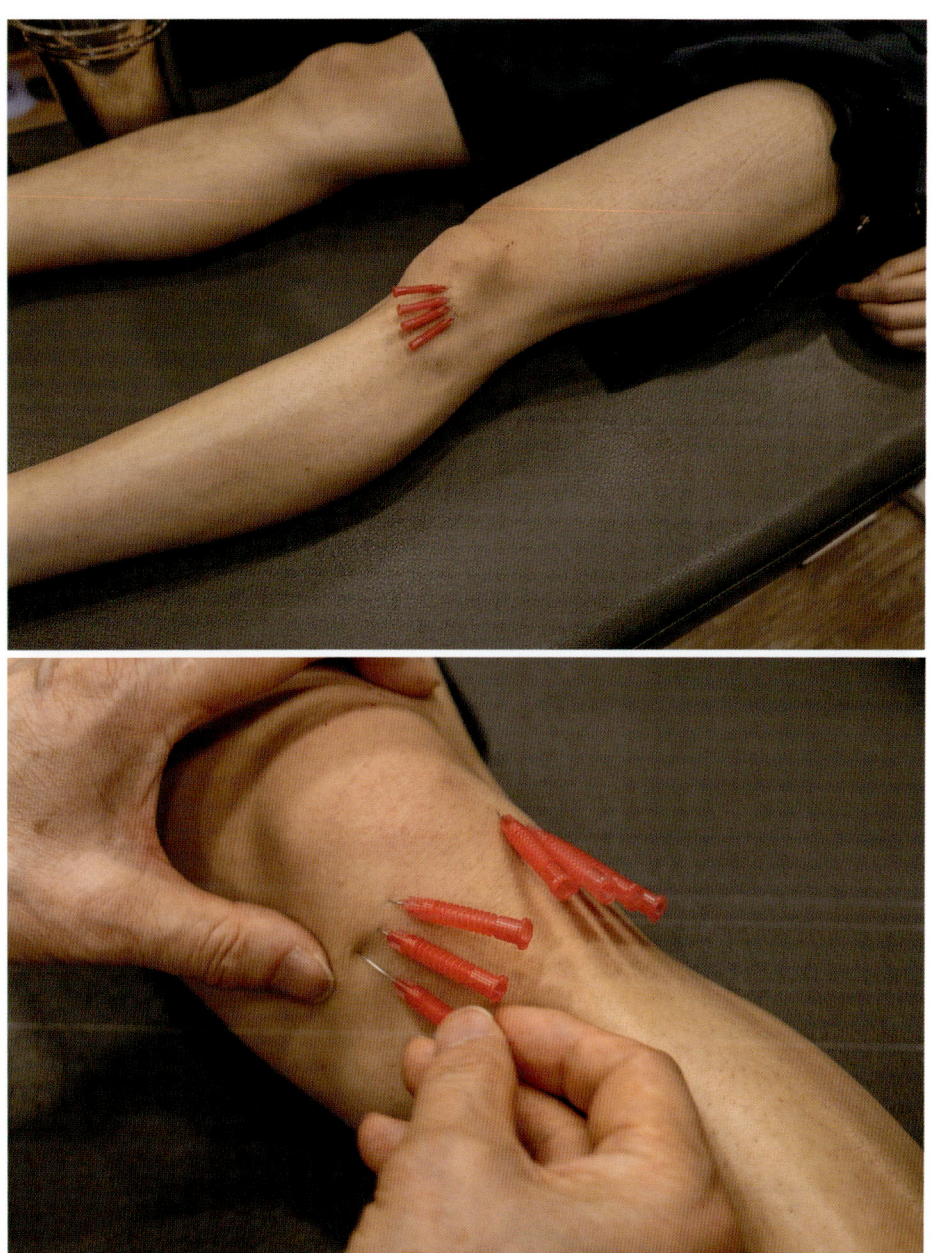

IV. Clinical Cases and Protocols

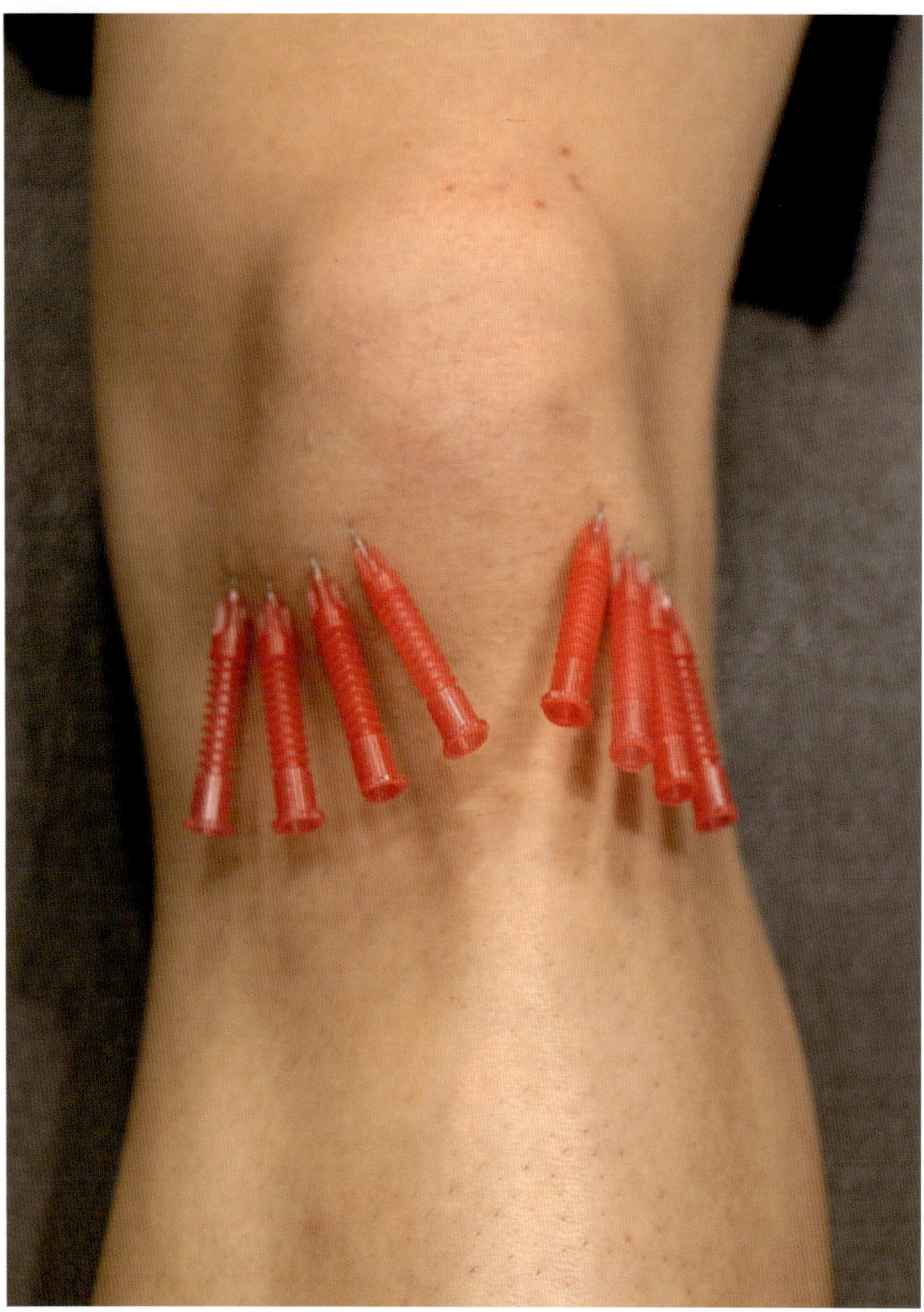

Insert threads transversely into the lateral retinaculum and medial retinaculum around the patella.

IV. Clinical Cases and Protocols

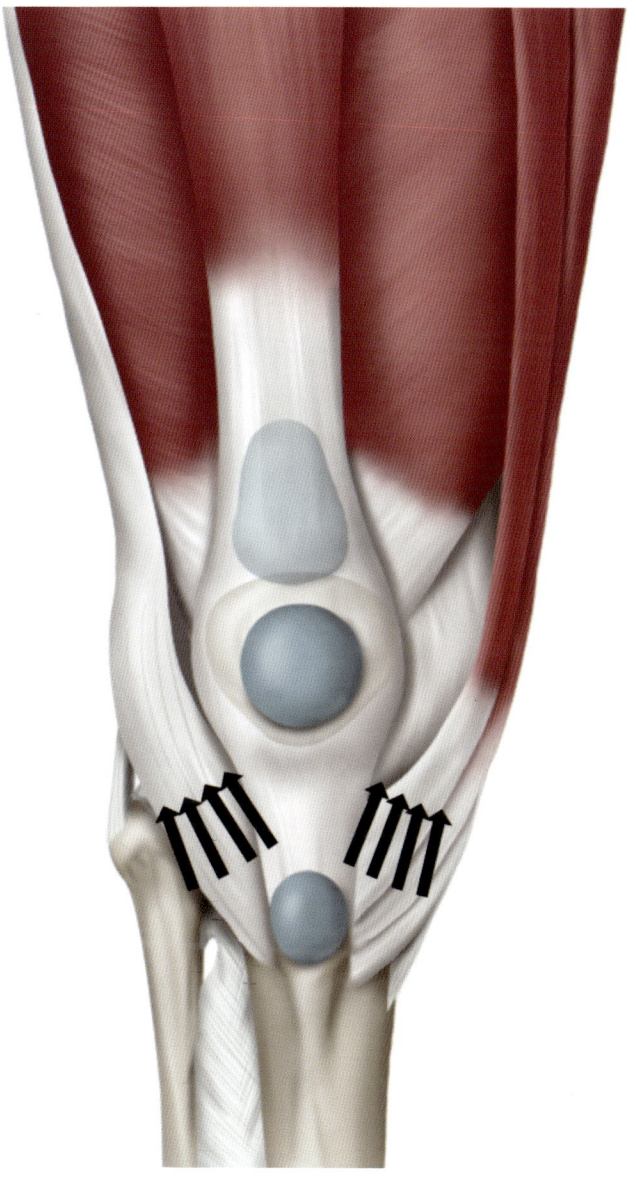

IV. Clinical Cases and Protocols

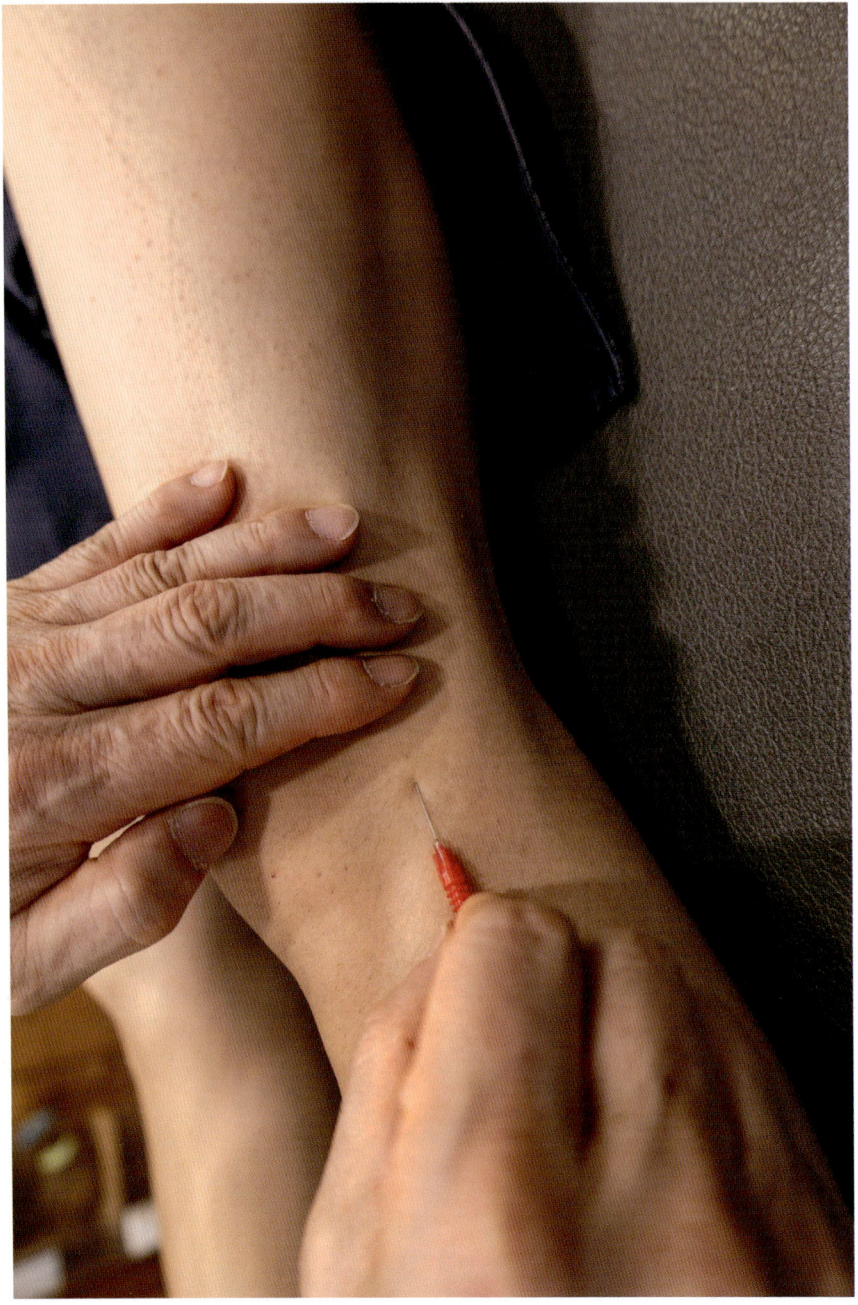

IV. Clinical Cases and Protocols

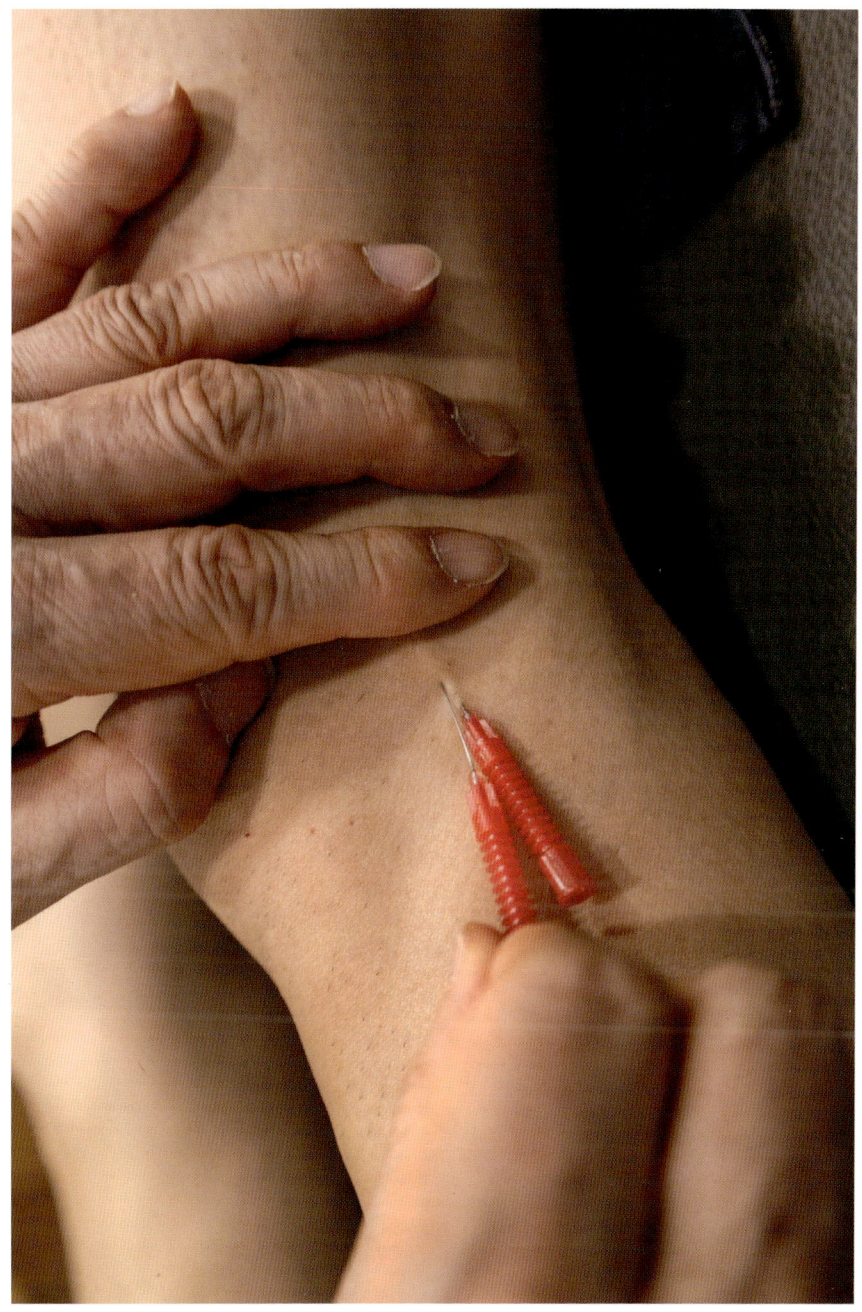

IV. Clinical Cases and Protocols

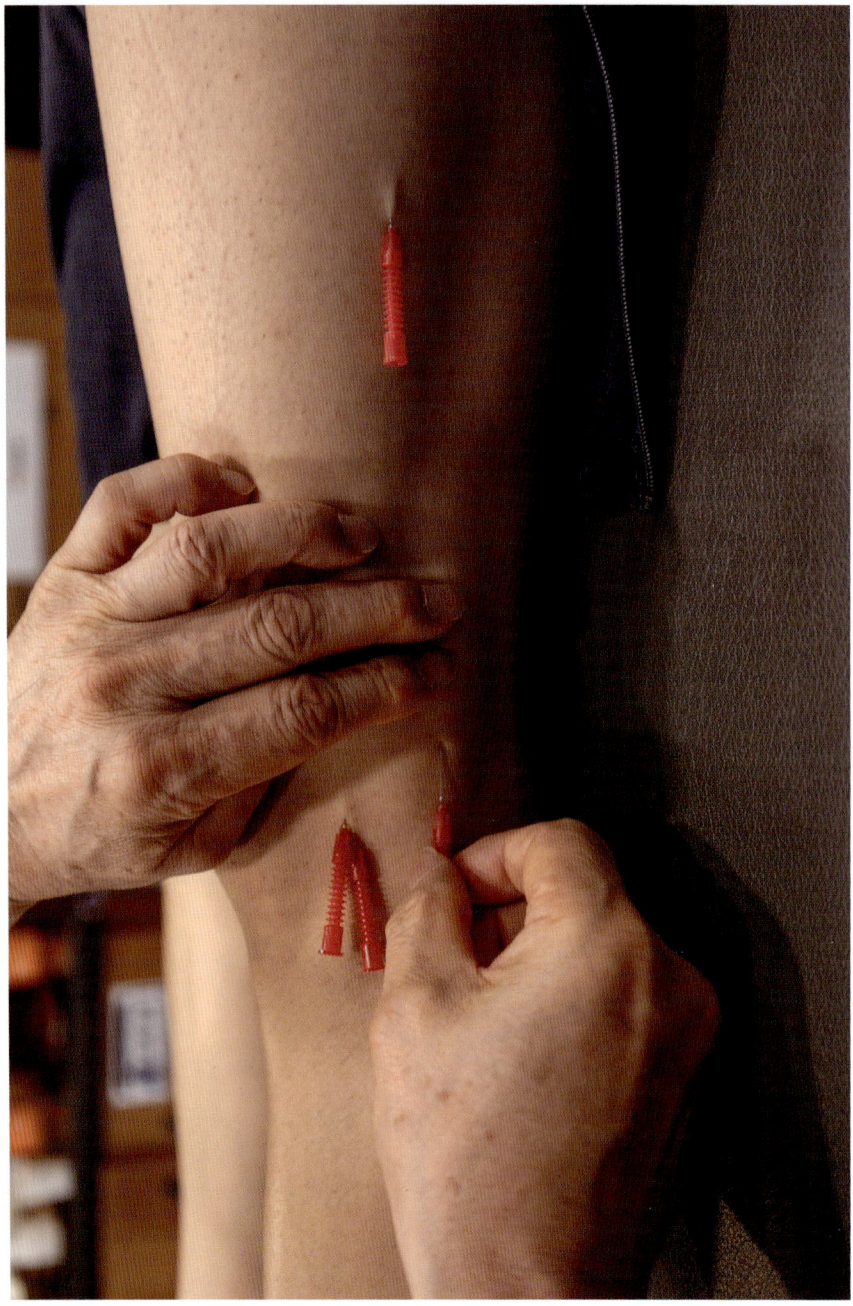

IV. Clinical Cases and Protocols

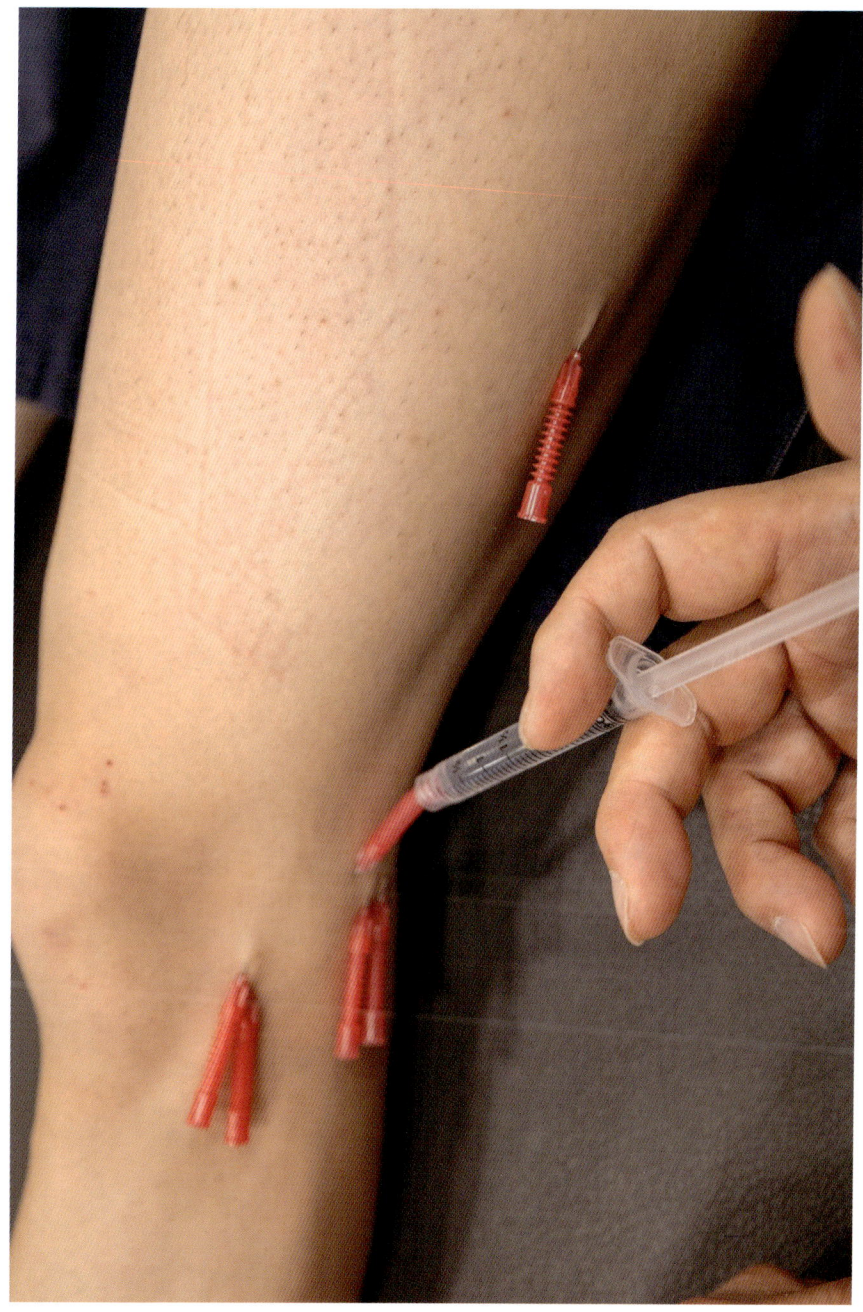

IV. Clinical Cases and Protocols

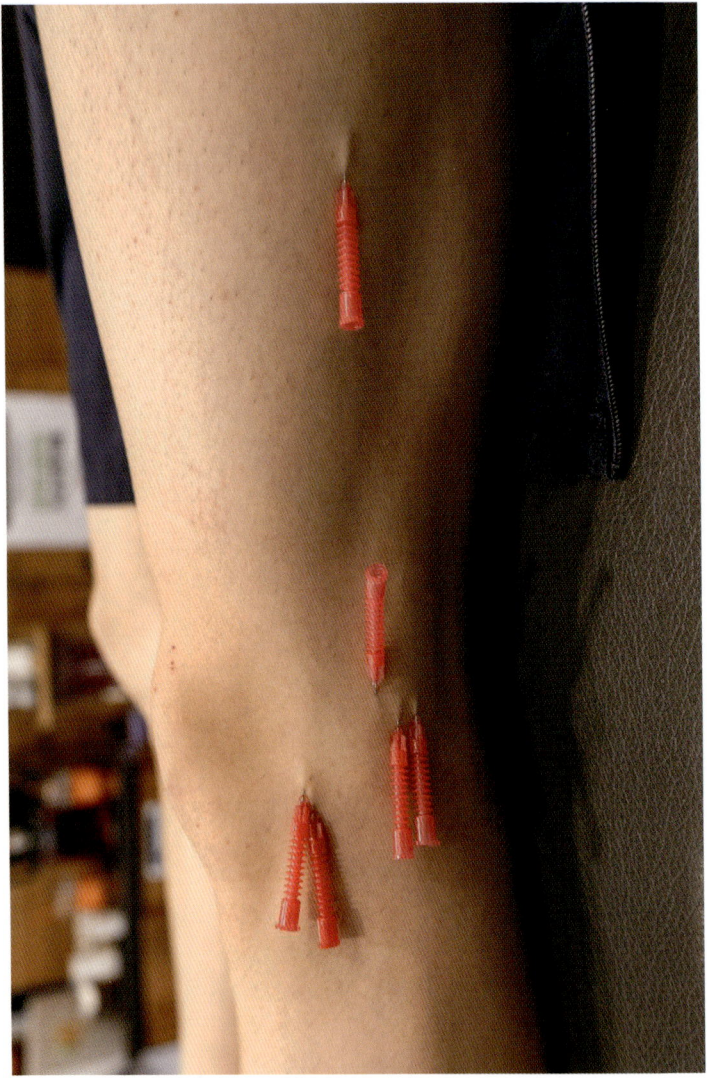

Insert threads transversely at the upper tibial attachment of the iliotibial band, specifically at the lateral condyle of the tibia (Gerdy's tubercle), and at the iliotibial band trigger point near Fengshi (風市, GB31).

Insert threads transversely at the fibular head, following the directions of the long head and short head of the biceps femoris, and administer pharmacopuncture.

Additionally, insert threads transversely along the lateral collateral ligament, and pharmacopuncture may be applied to this area as well.

IV. Clinical Cases and Protocols

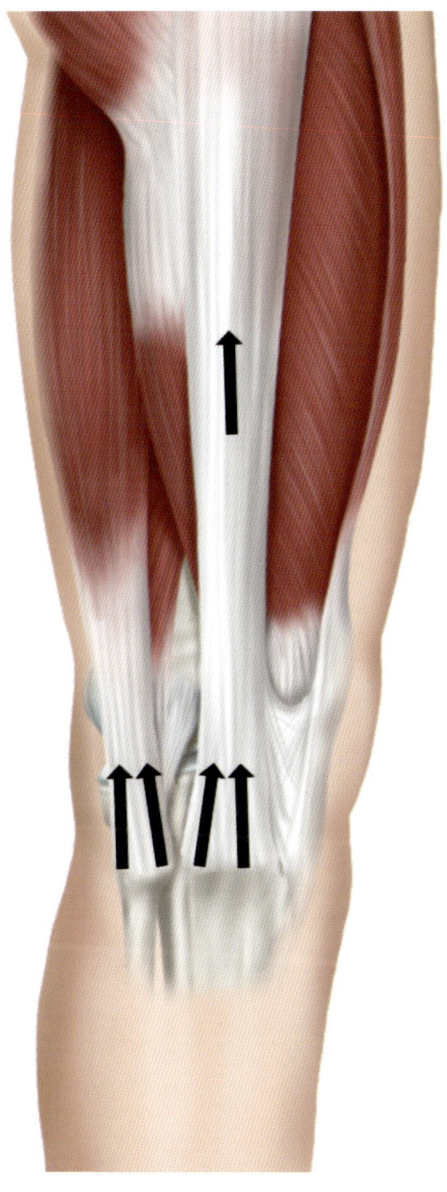

IV. Clinical Cases and Protocols

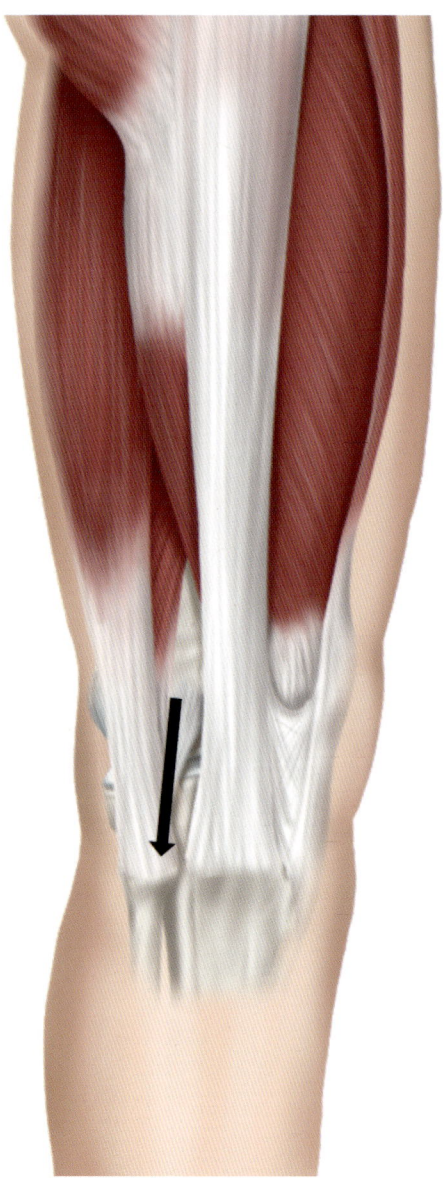

IV. Clinical Cases and Protocols

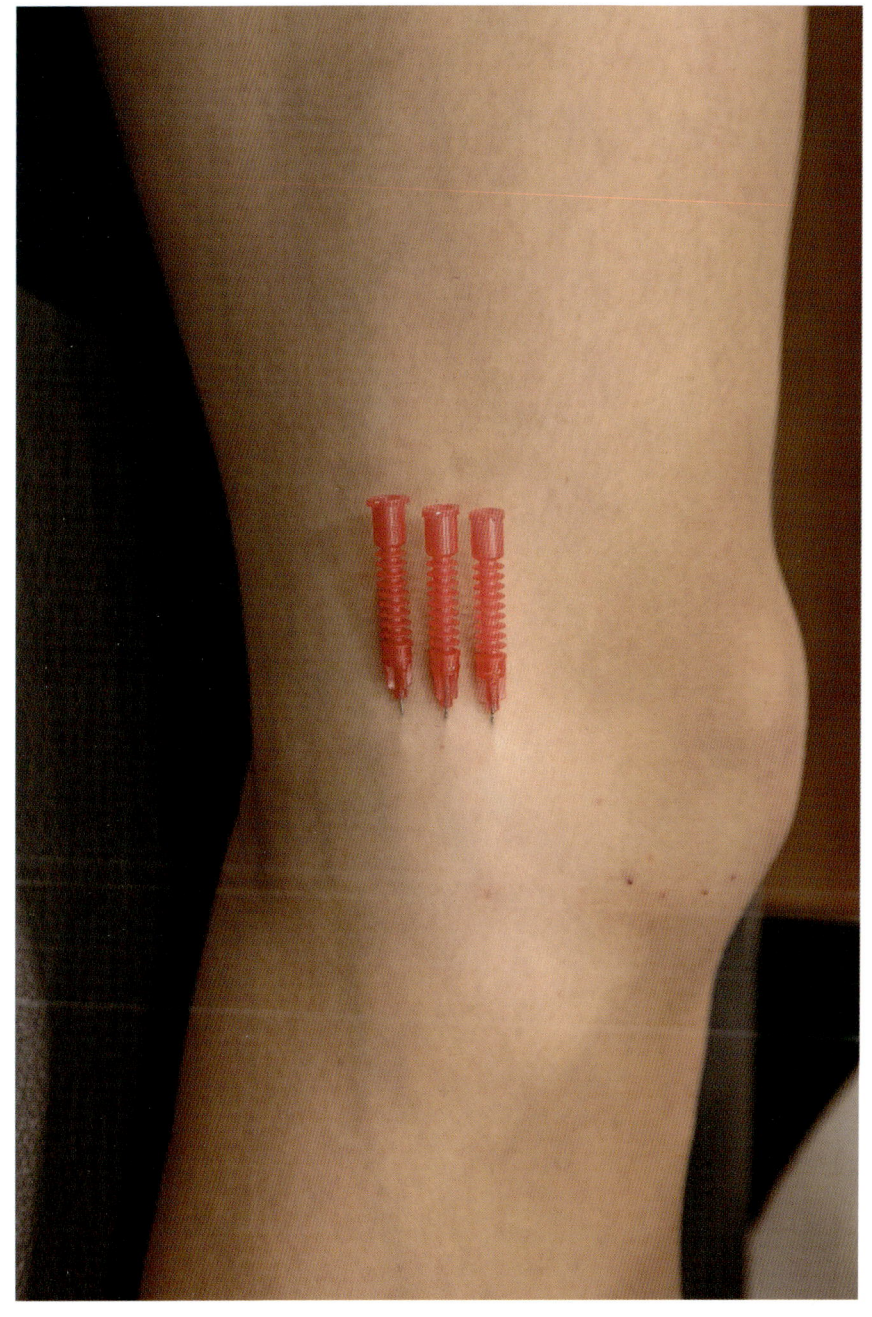

IV. Clinical Cases and Protocols

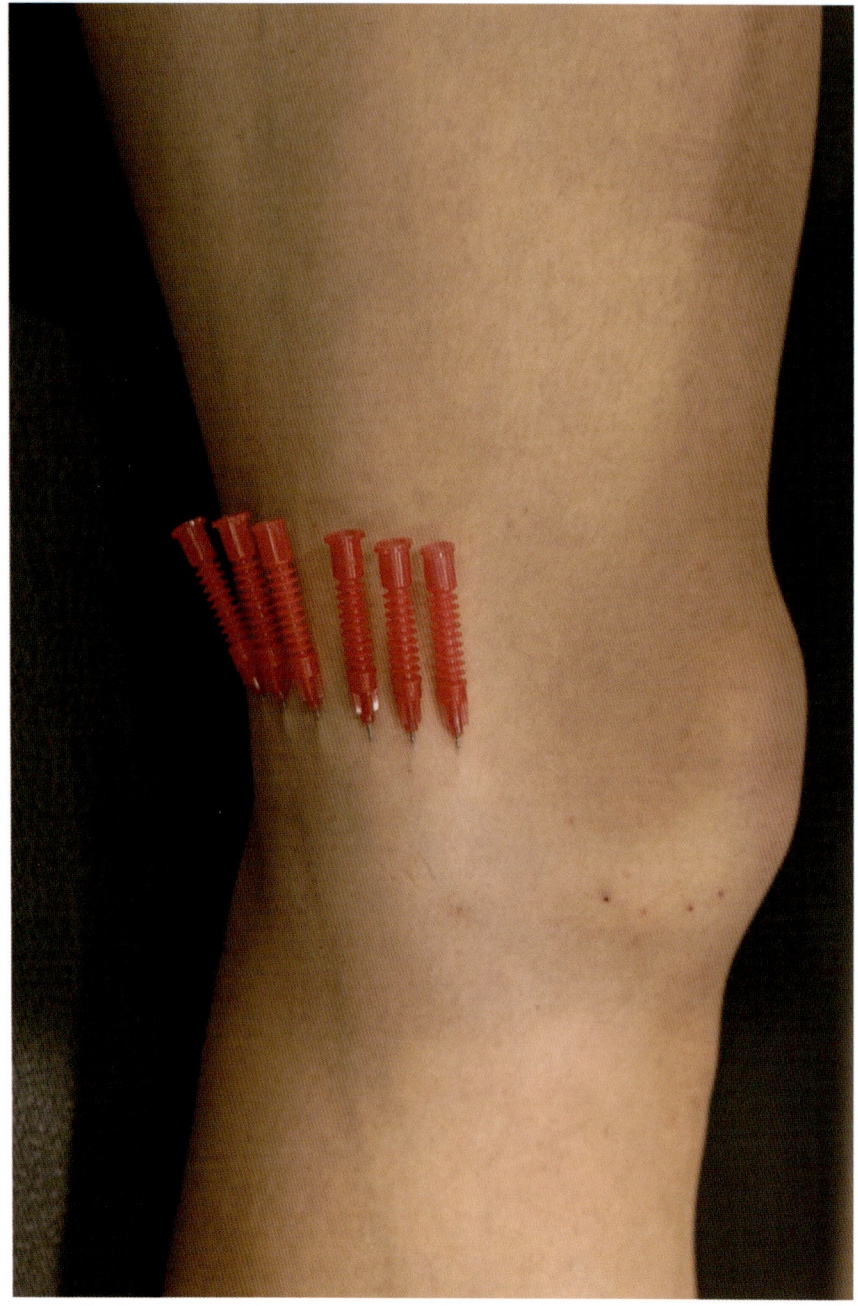

IV. Clinical Cases and Protocols

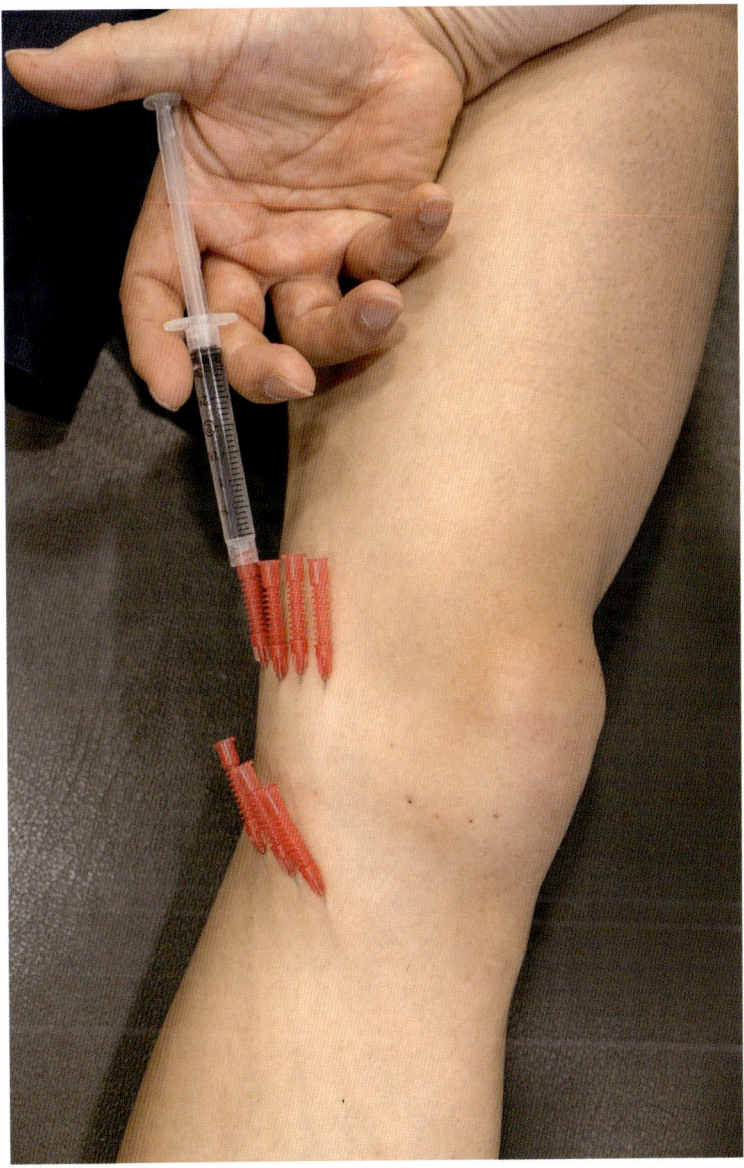

Insert threads transversely into the sartorius, gracilis, semimembranosus, and semitendinosus muscles.

For the pes anserine bursa, insert threads transversely at the medial tibial attachment of the sartorius, gracilis, and semitendinosus muscles, and administer pharmacopuncture at the same sites.

IV. Clinical Cases and Protocols

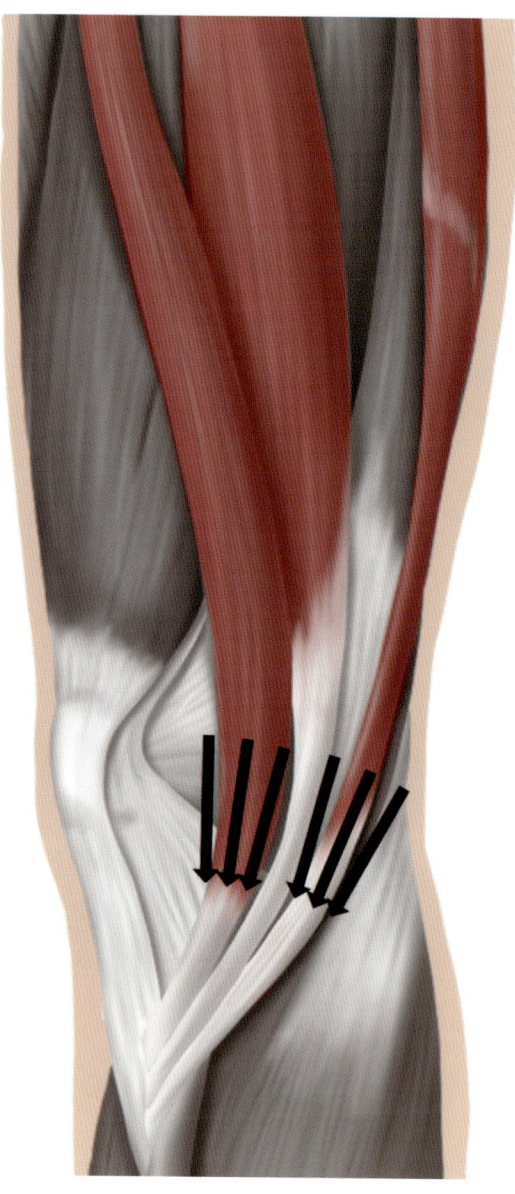

IV. Clinical Cases and Protocols

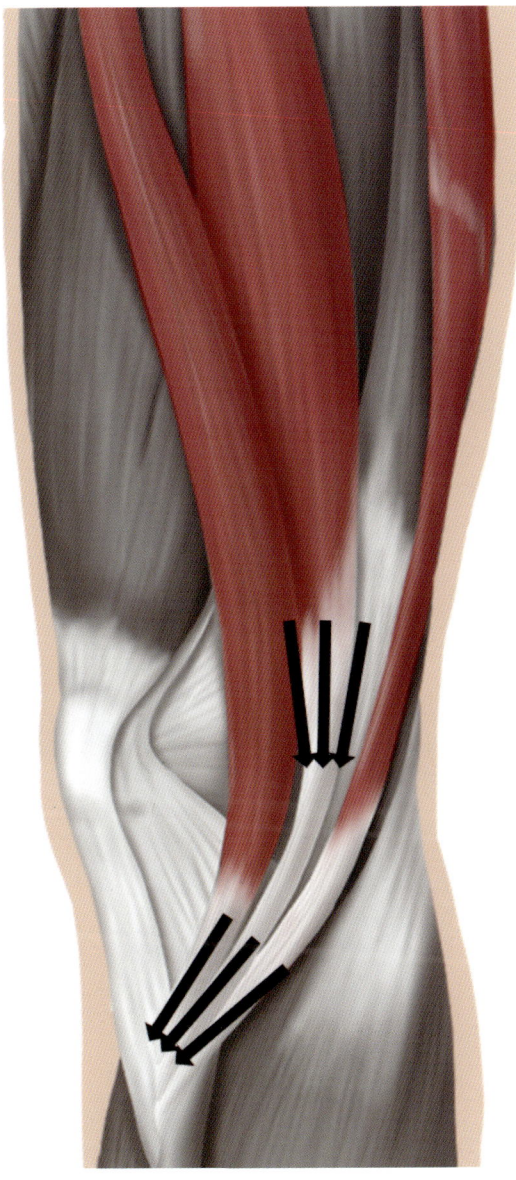

IV. Clinical Cases and Protocols

Posterior thigh muscles

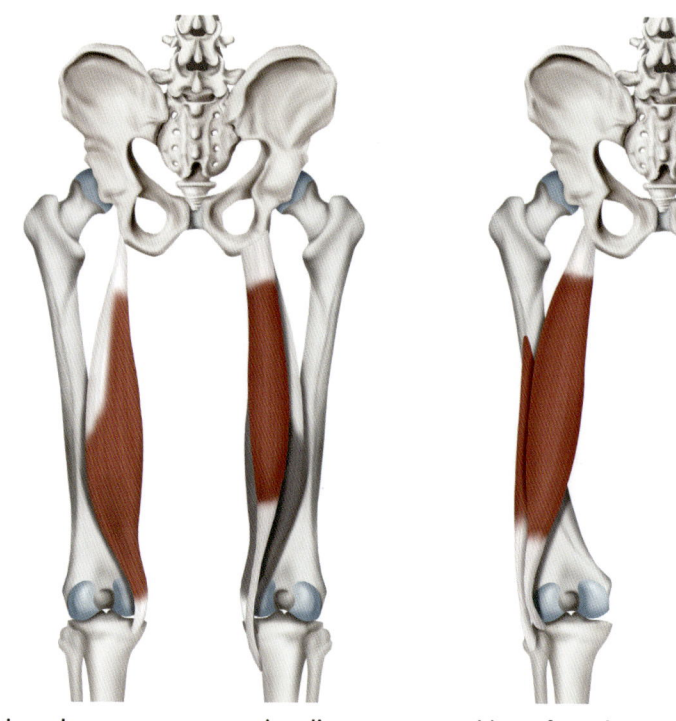

semimembranosus m. semitendinosus m. biceps femoris m. hamstring

IV. Clinical Cases and Protocols

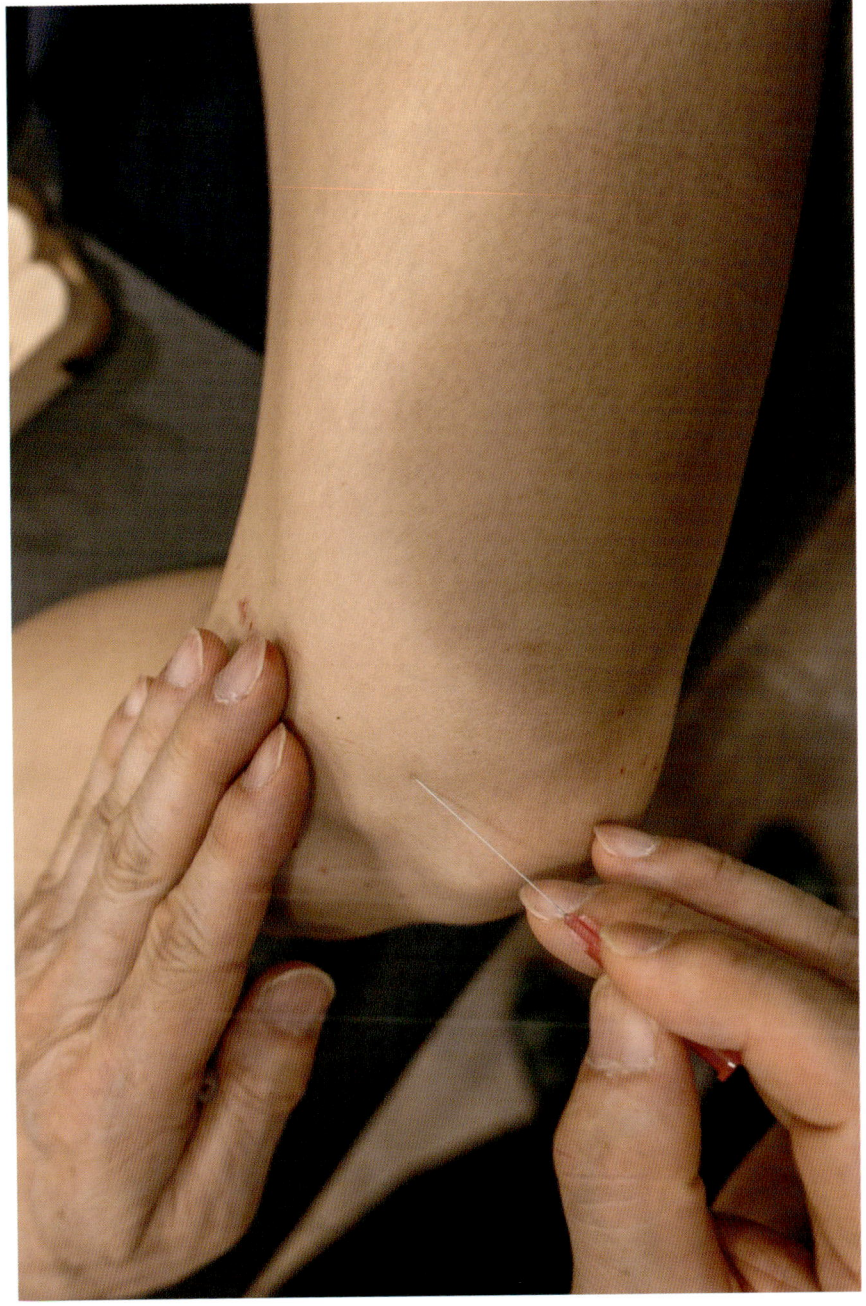

IV. Clinical Cases and Protocols

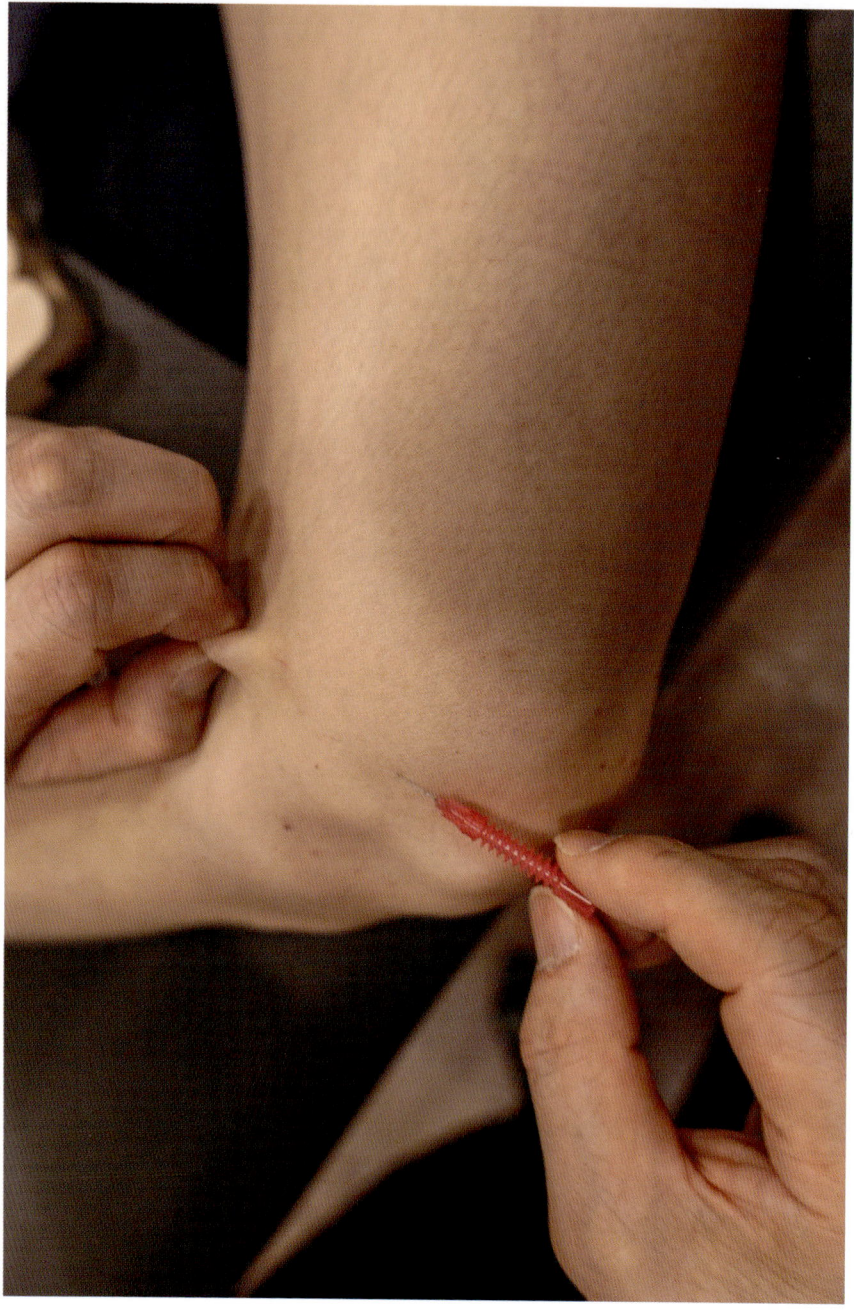

IV. Clinical Cases and Protocols

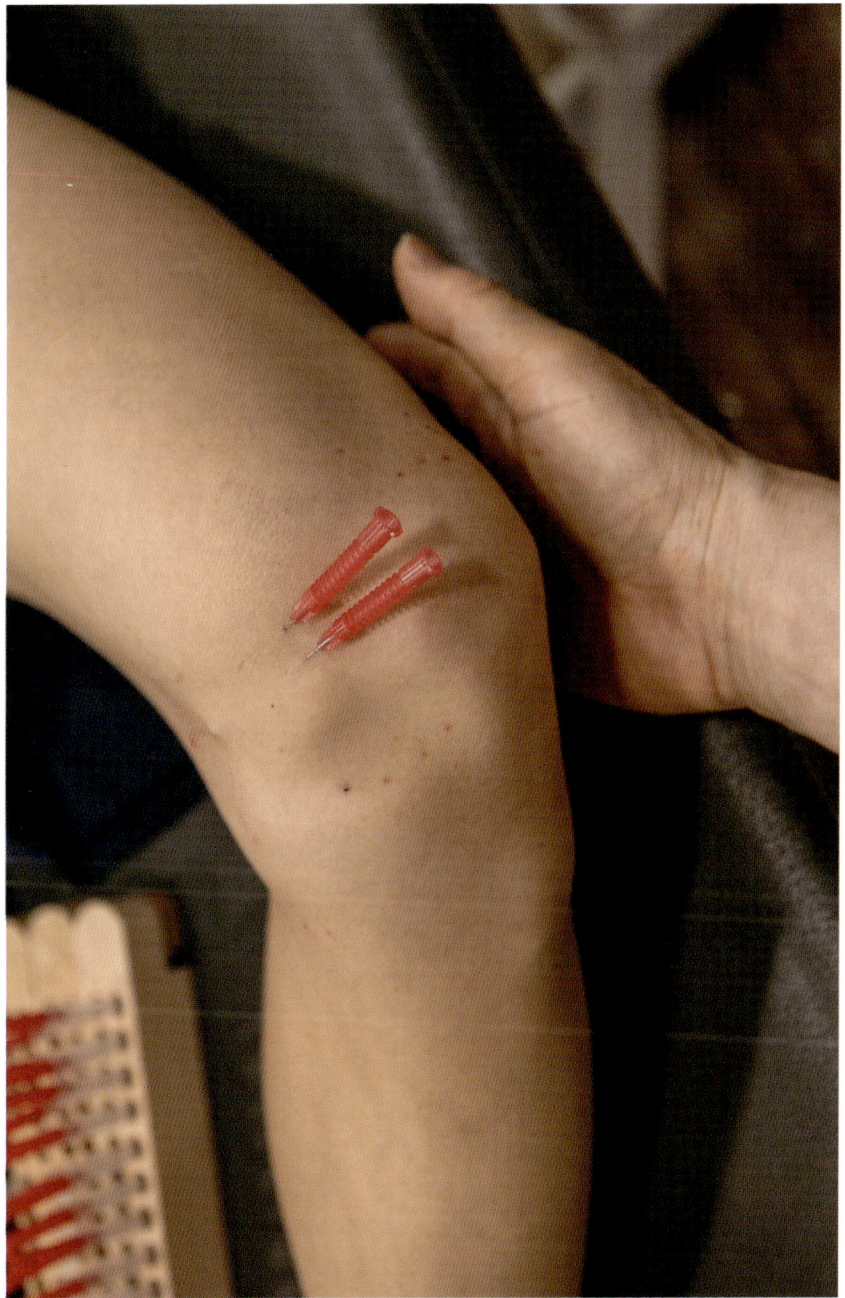

Perform a crosshatch pattern of thread embedding extending to the areas of the medial collateral ligament and the medial patellofemoral ligament.

IV. Clinical Cases and Protocols

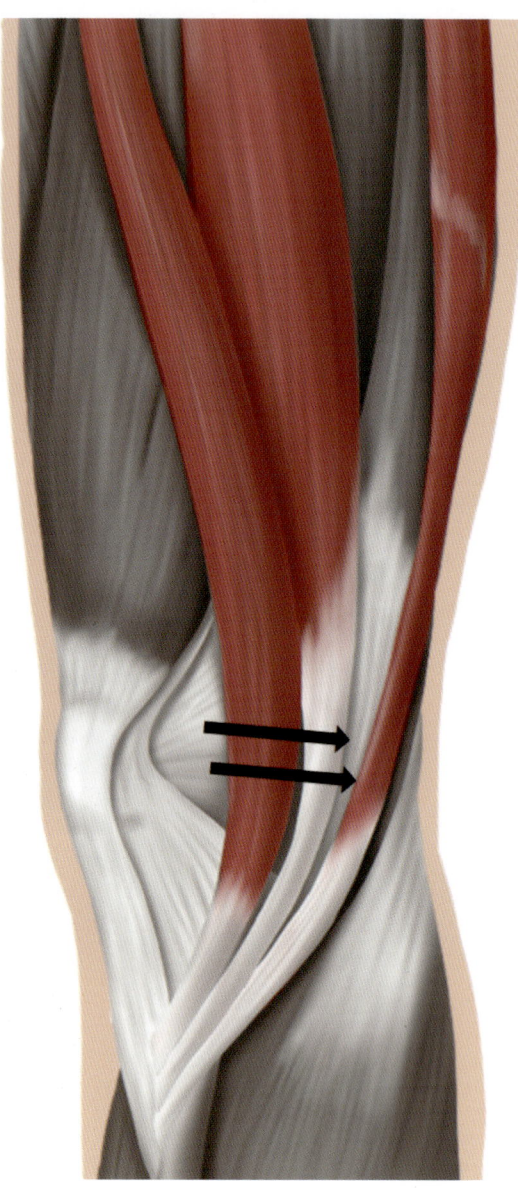

IV. Clinical Cases and Protocols

4. Ankle Joint

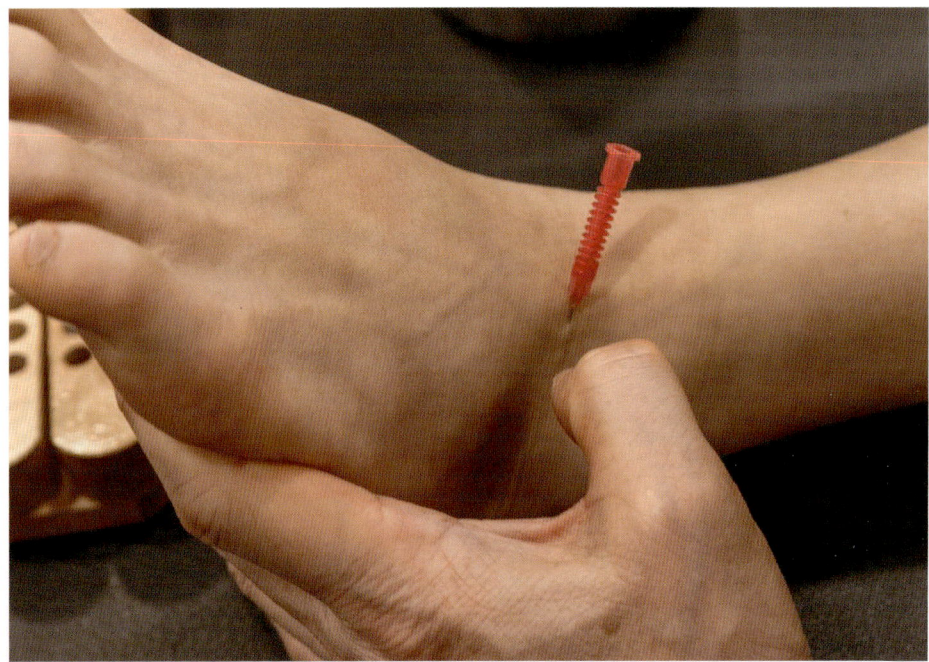

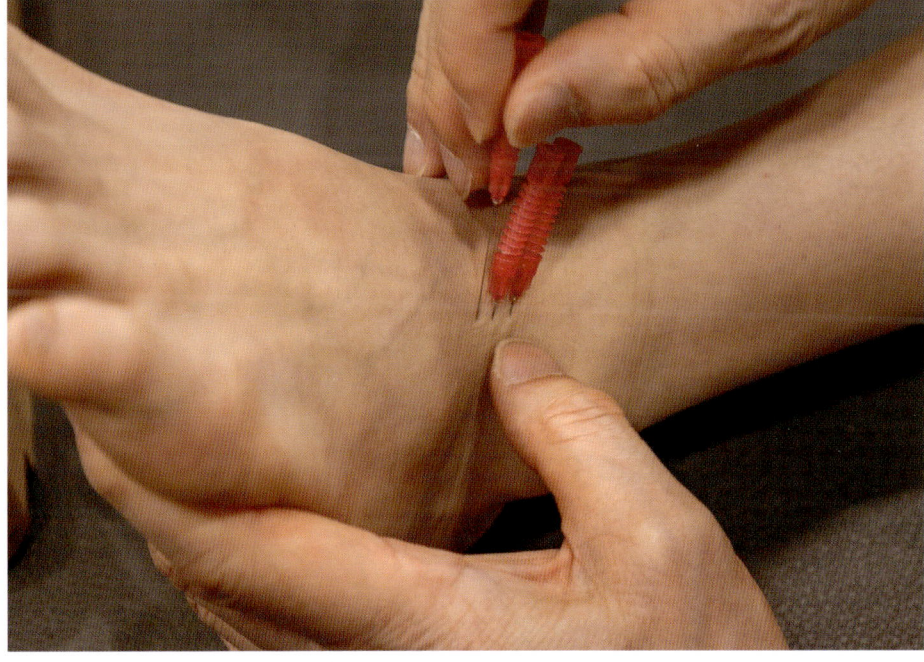

IV. Clinical Cases and Protocols

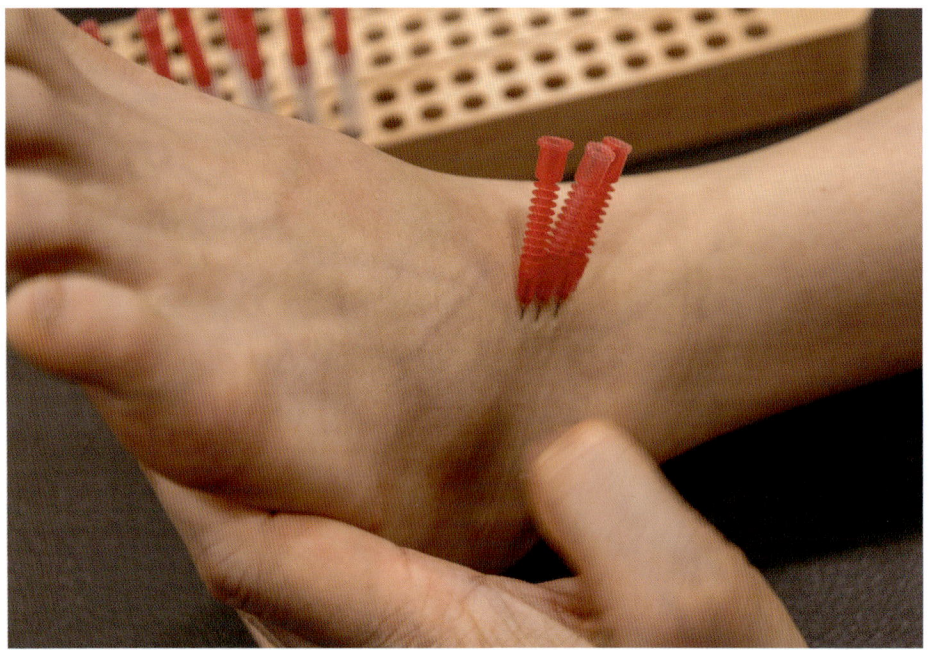

Insert threads transversely into the inferior extensor retinaculum.

IV. Clinical Cases and Protocols

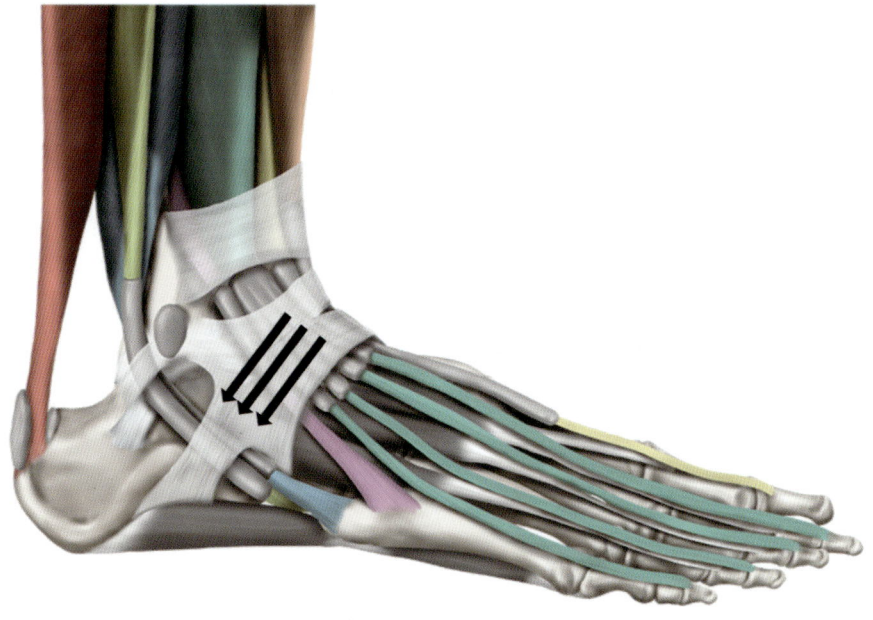

IV. Clinical Cases and Protocols

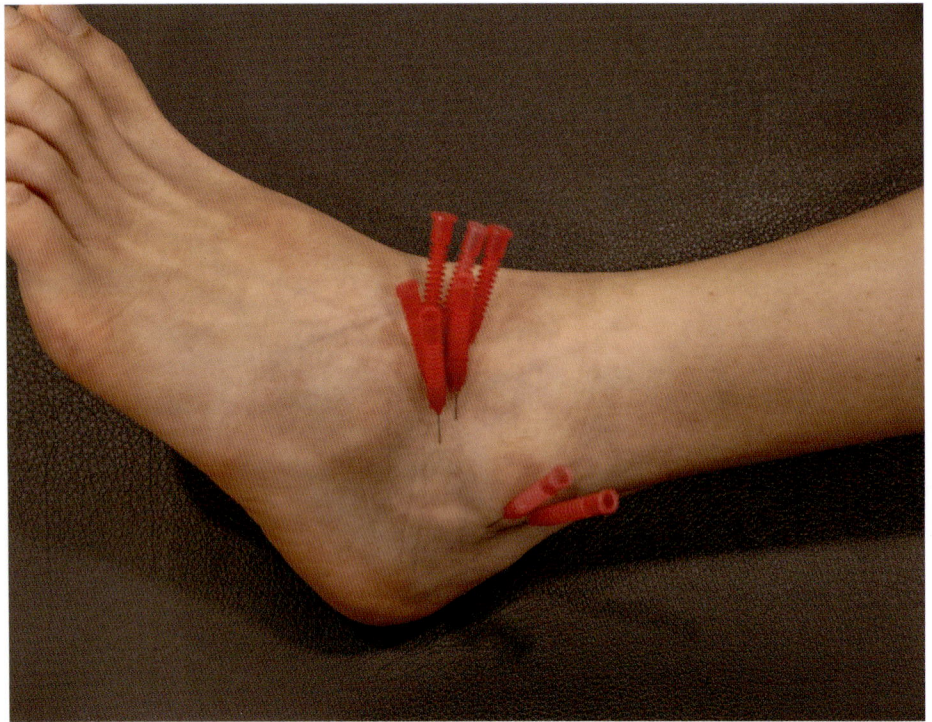

Insert threads transversely into the superior peroneal retinaculum.

IV. Clinical Cases and Protocols

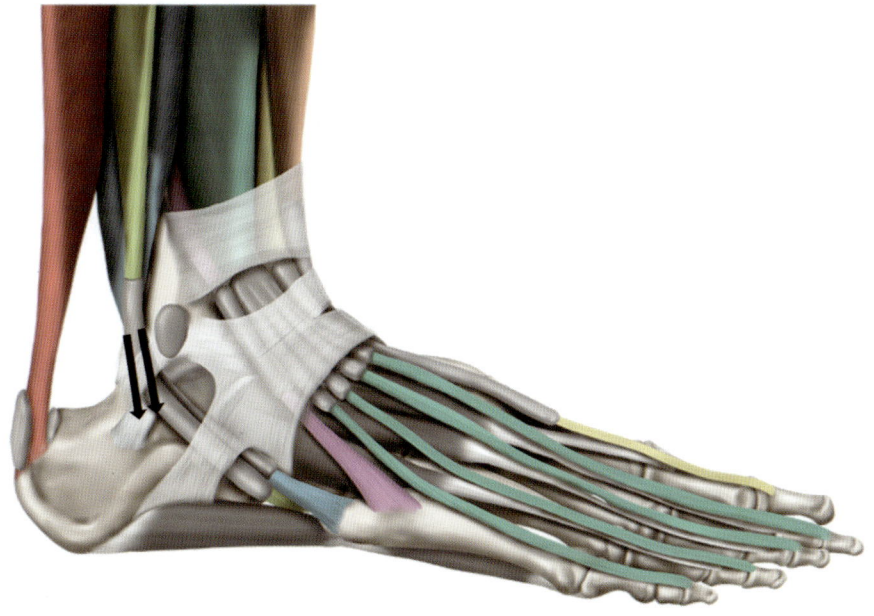

IV. Clinical Cases and Protocols

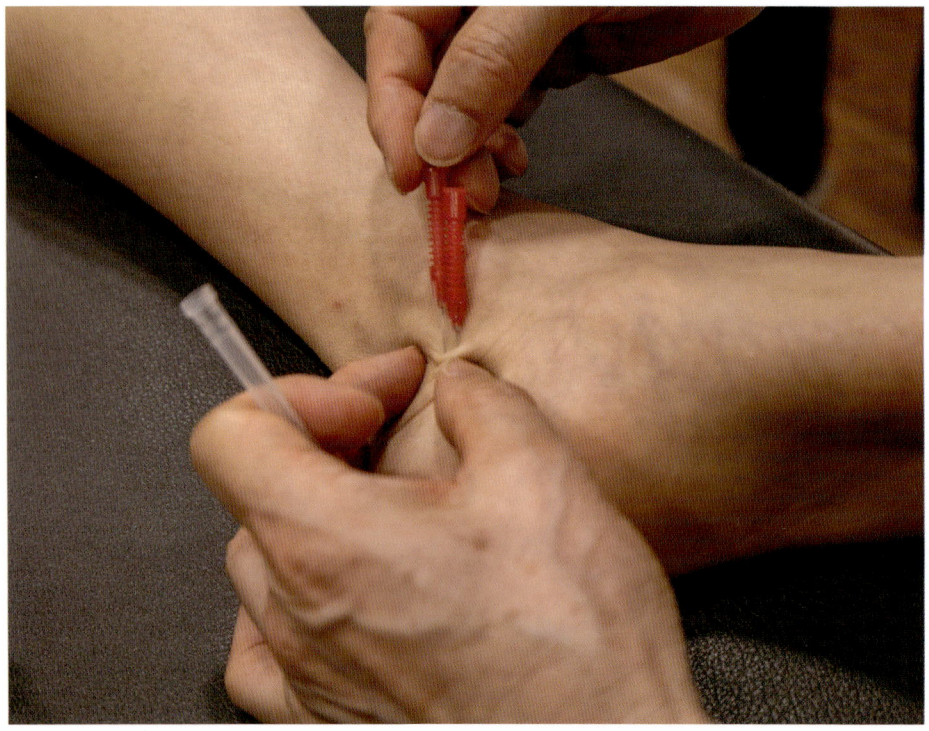

Insert threads transversely into the flexor retinaculum, directing the insertion toward its attachment on the calcaneus.

IV. Clinical Cases and Protocols

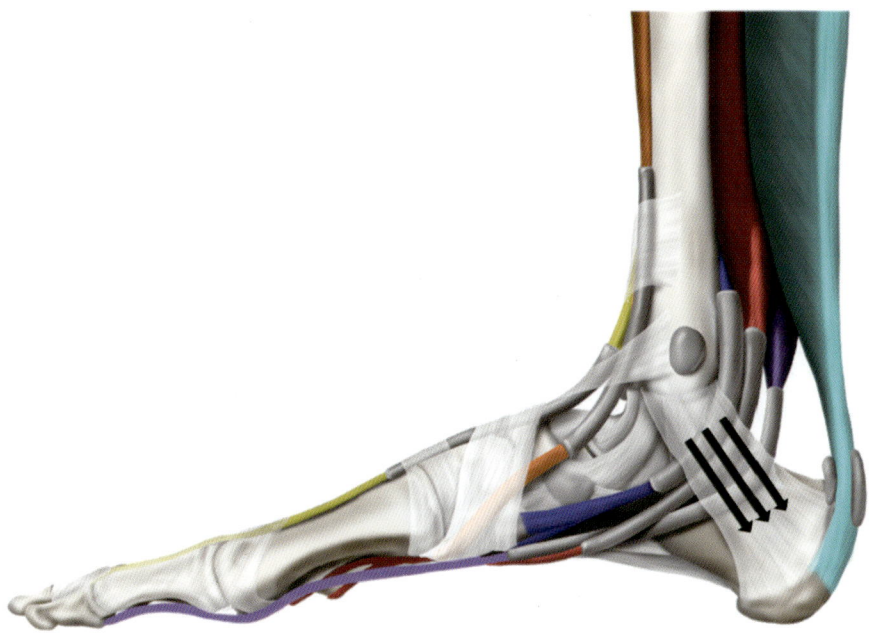

IV. Clinical Cases and Protocols

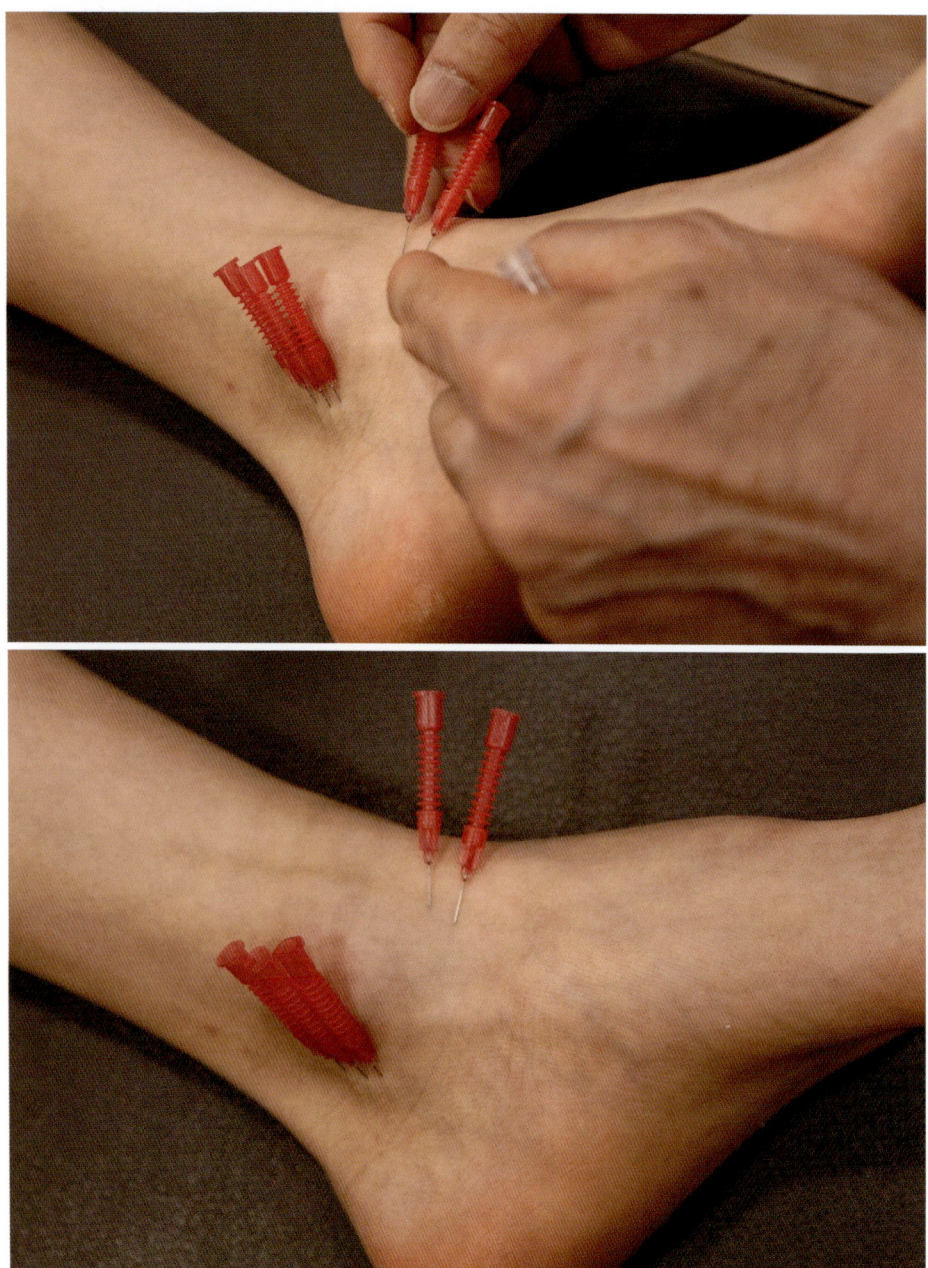

Insert threads transversely into the medial portion of the inferior extensor retinaculum.

IV. Clinical Cases and Protocols

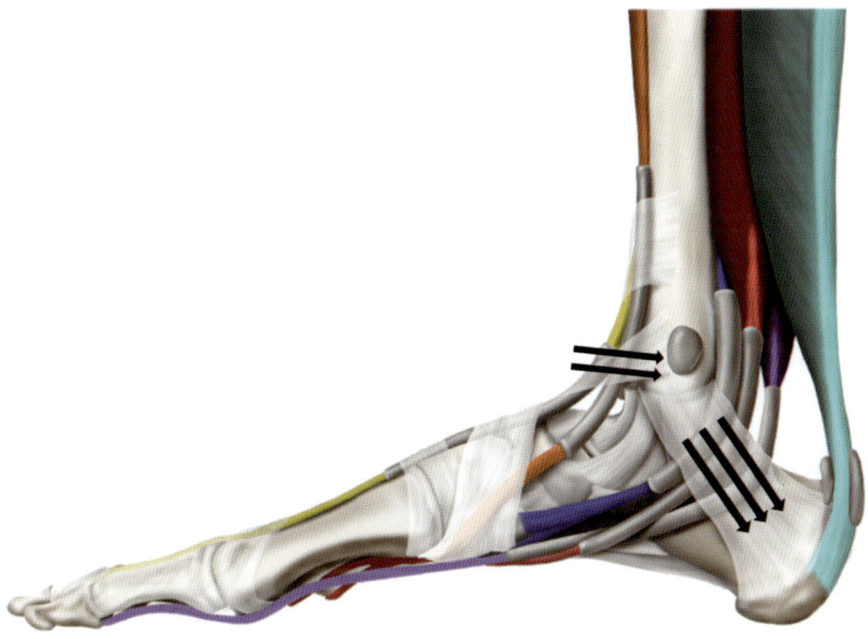

IV. Clinical Cases and Protocols

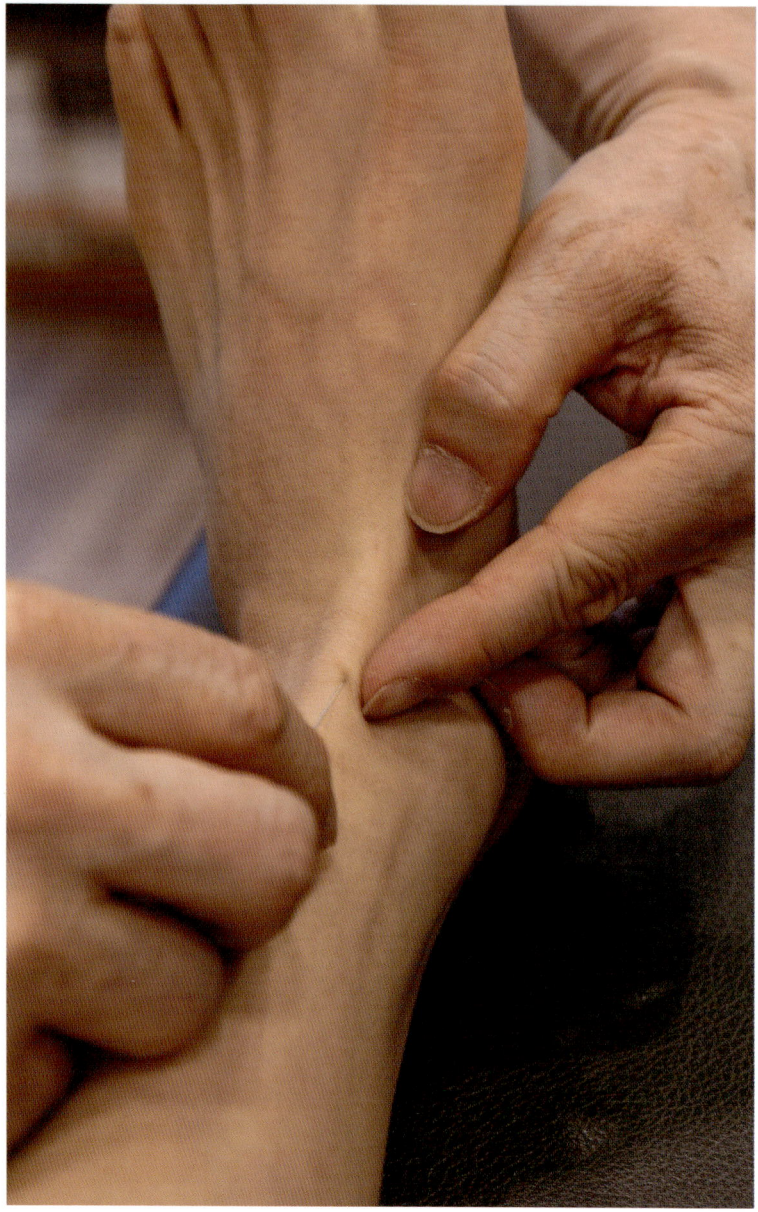

IV. Clinical Cases and Protocols

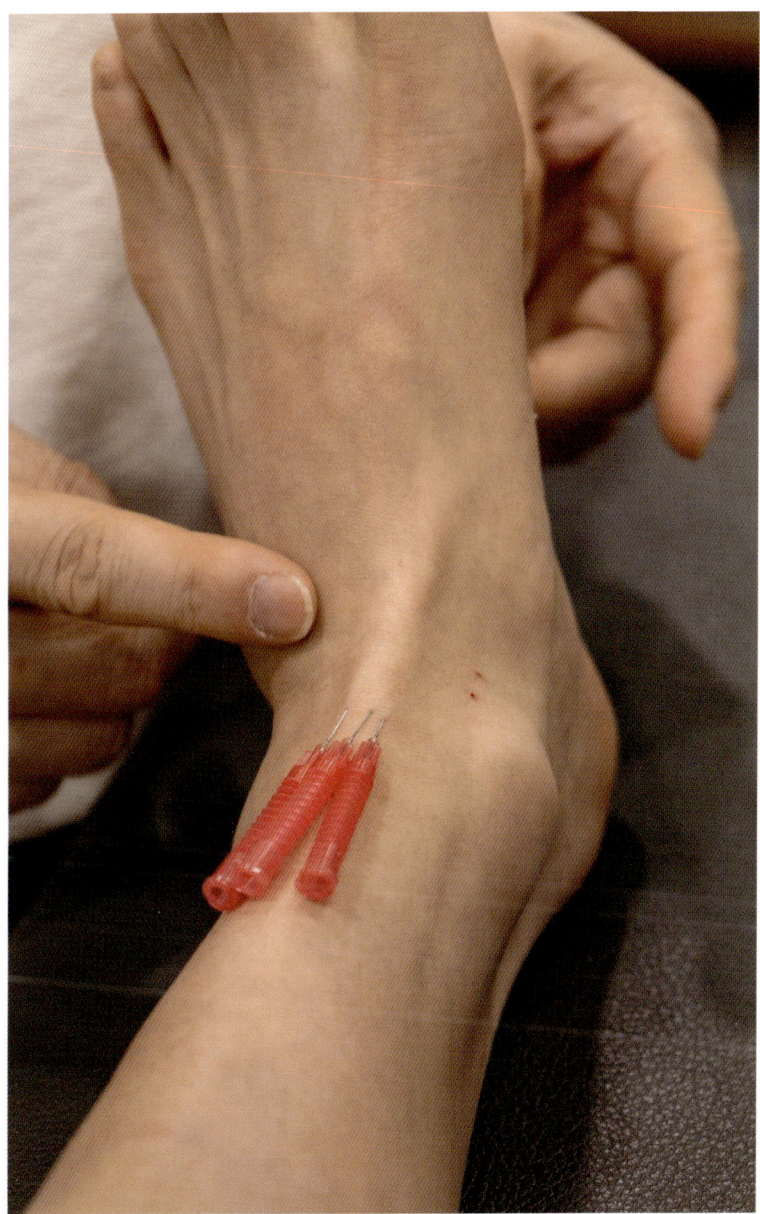

When a specific muscle is identified as the source of the problem, diagnose the precise point of dysfunction and insert threads transversely at the target site.
For example, in cases involving the extensor hallucis longus, threads can be inserted transversely as shown in the accompanying image.

IV. Clinical Cases and Protocols

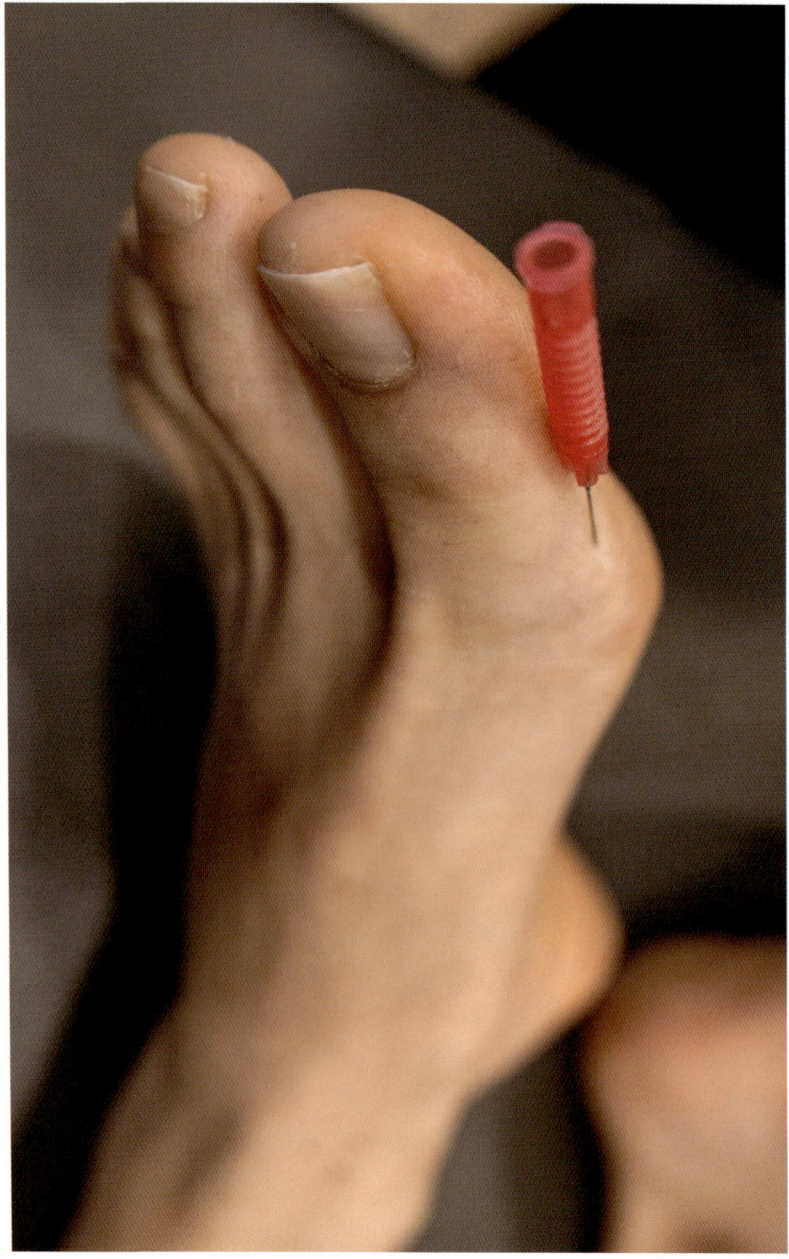

IV. Clinical Cases and Protocols

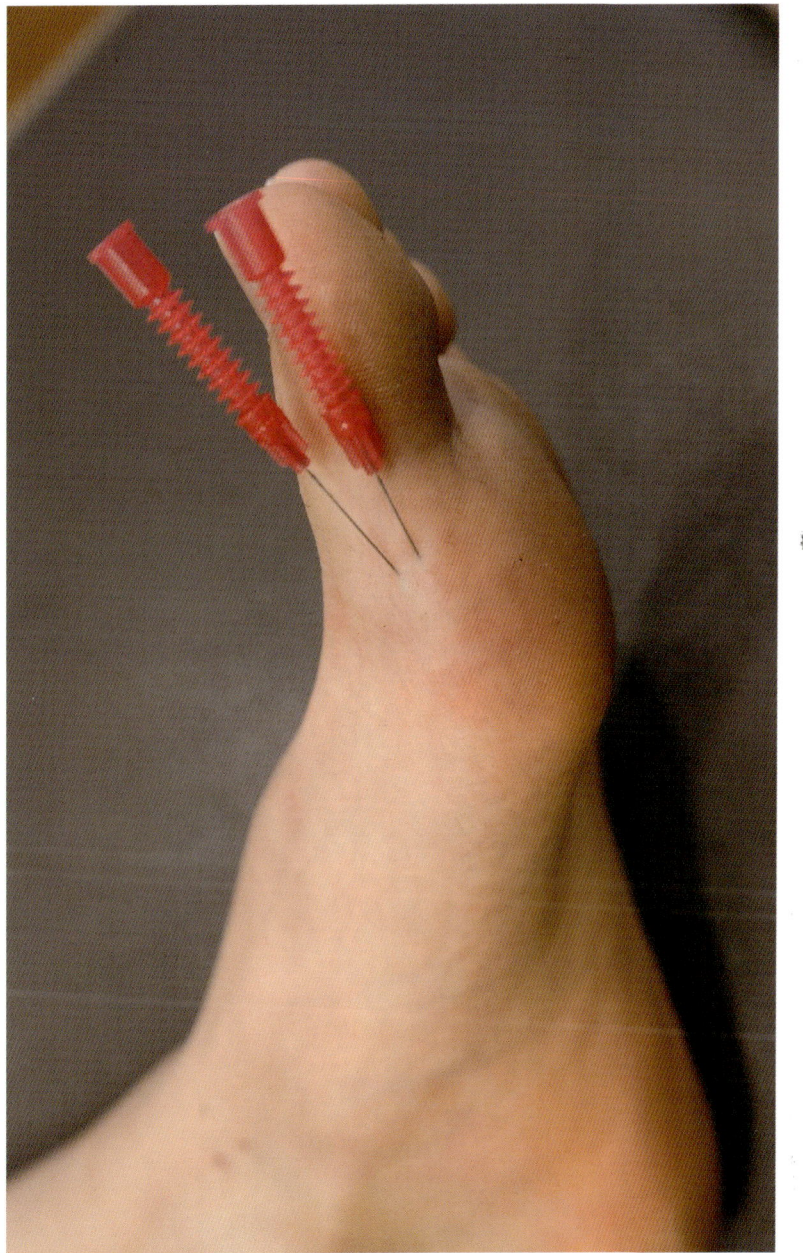

Thread embedding can also be applied transversely to the abductor hallucis tendon, which is commonly involved in cases of hallux valgus, as part of the treatment approach.

IV. Clinical Cases and Protocols

5. Shoulder Joint

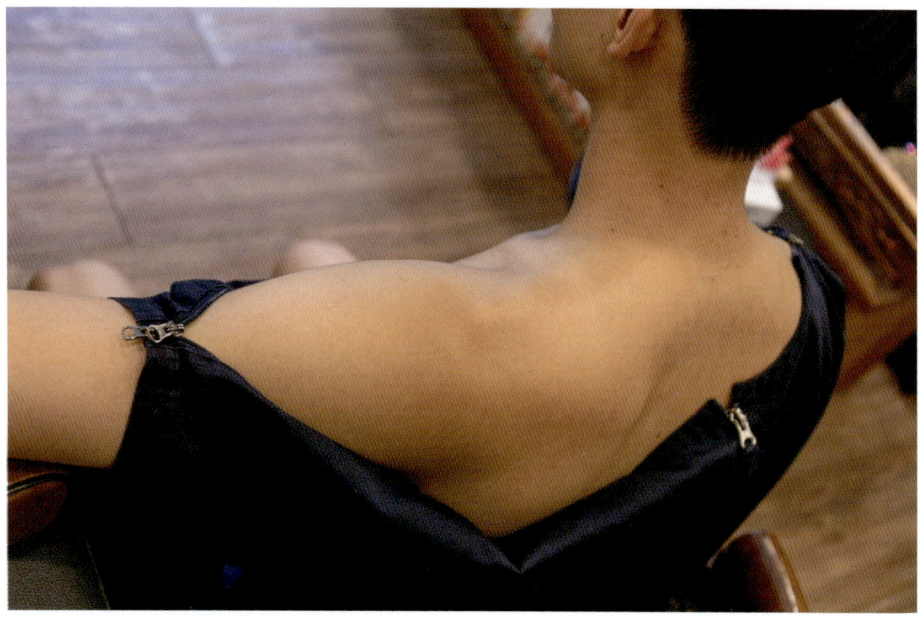

For thread embedding treatment of the shoulder joint, it is recommended to perform the procedure with the patient in a seated position and the affected arm raised to shoulder height.

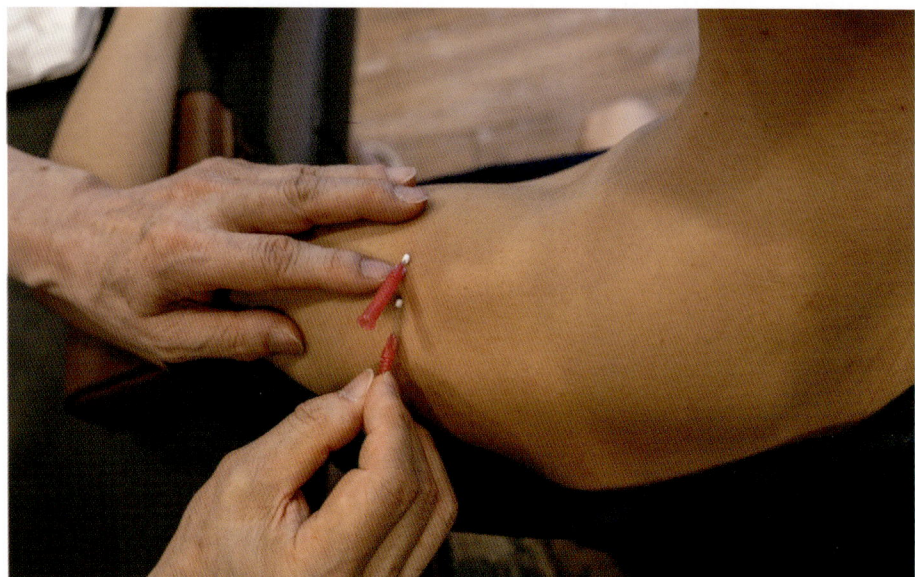

IV. Clinical Cases and Protocols

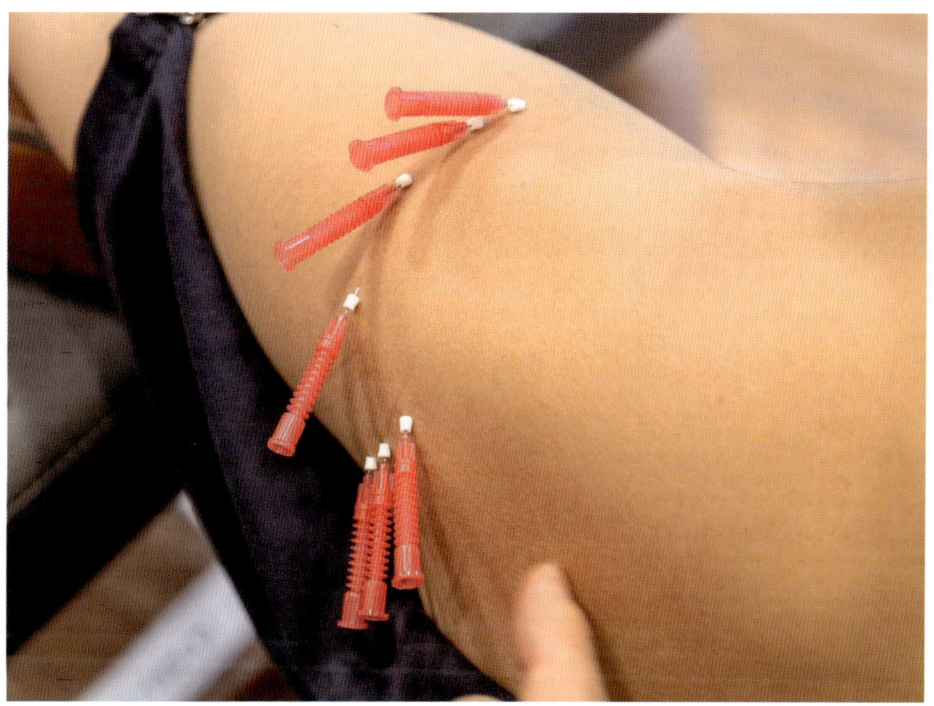

Insert threads transversely around the origin of the deltoid muscle—including the lateral third of the clavicle, the acromion, and the inferior edge of the scapular spine.
Also, insert threads transversely into the teres minor muscle.

IV. Clinical Cases and Protocols

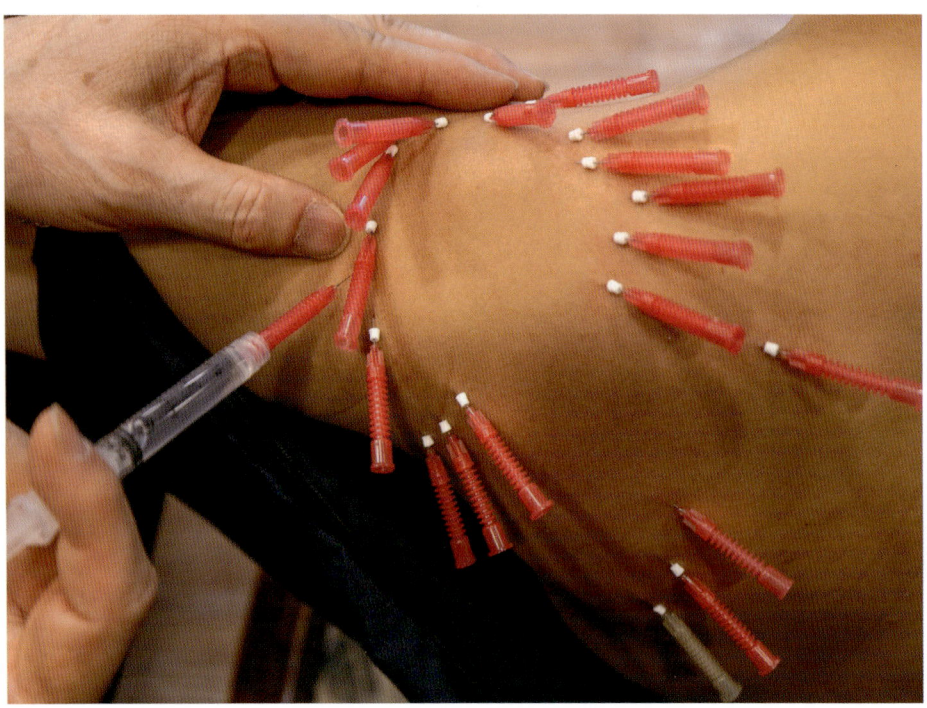

Below the origin of the deltoid muscle, target the area above the subacromial bursa, and perform thread embedding and pharmacopuncture simultaneously, wrapping around the rotator cuff.

IV. Clinical Cases and Protocols

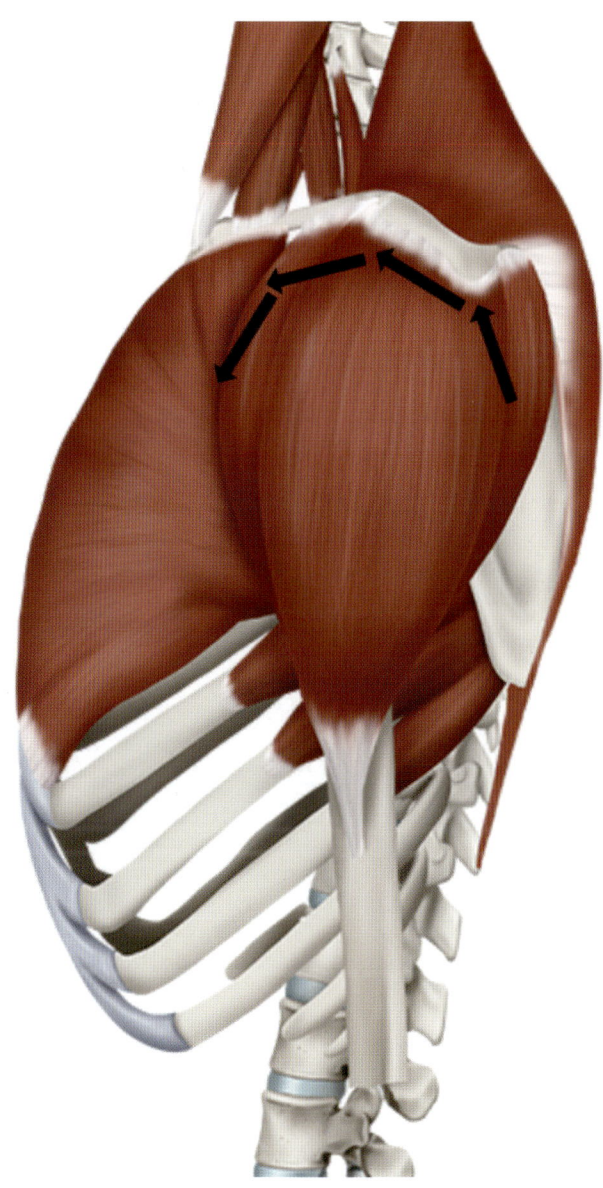

Thread embedding is performed encircling the deltoid muscle.

IV. Clinical Cases and Protocols

Shoulder Anatomy

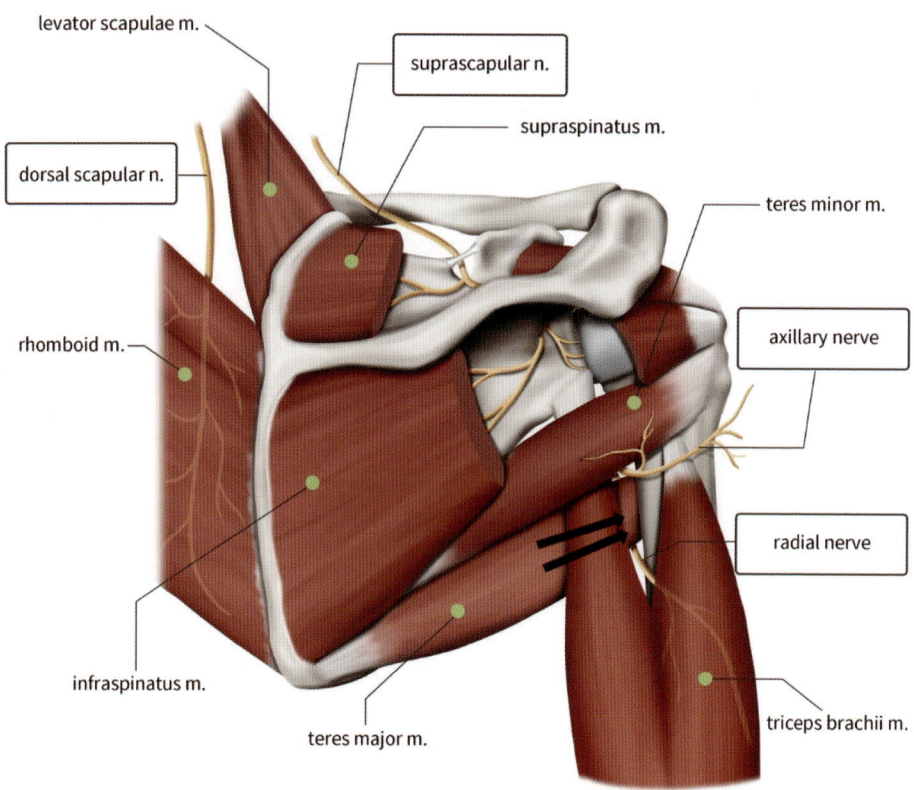

IV. Clinical Cases and Protocols

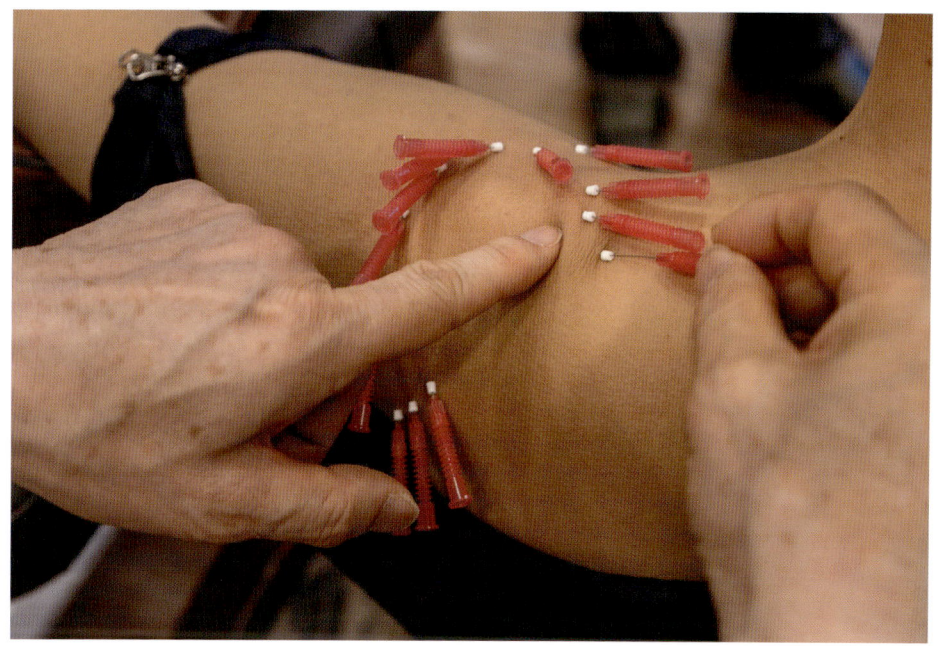

For the supraspinatus muscle, insert the thread parallel to the muscle fibers, just below the acromion.

Perform thread embedding and pharmacopuncture simultaneously over the subacromial bursa.

IV. Clinical Cases and Protocols

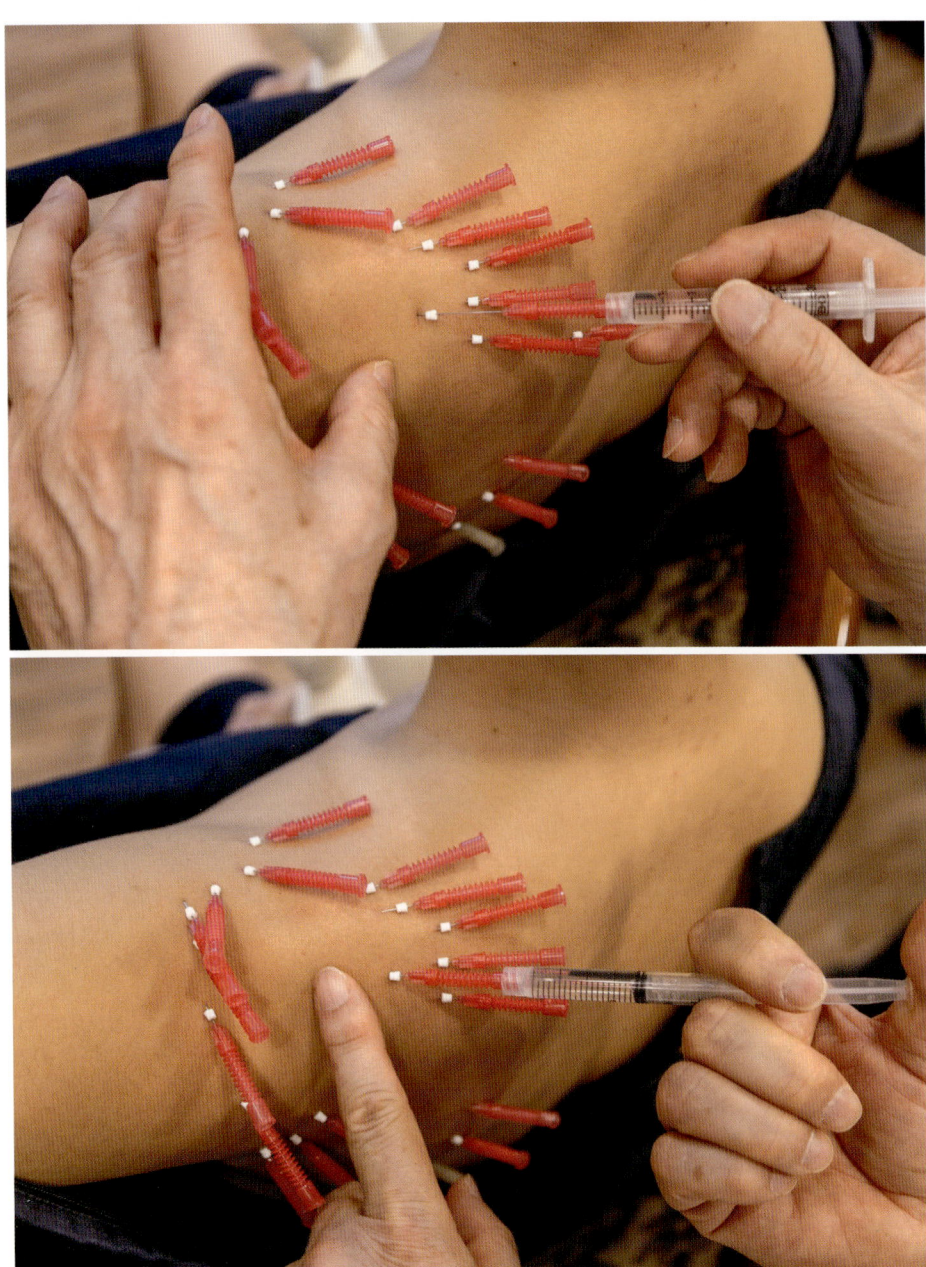

Administering pharmacopuncture in addition to thread embedding beneath the acromion can further enhance therapeutic effectiveness.

IV. Clinical Cases and Protocols

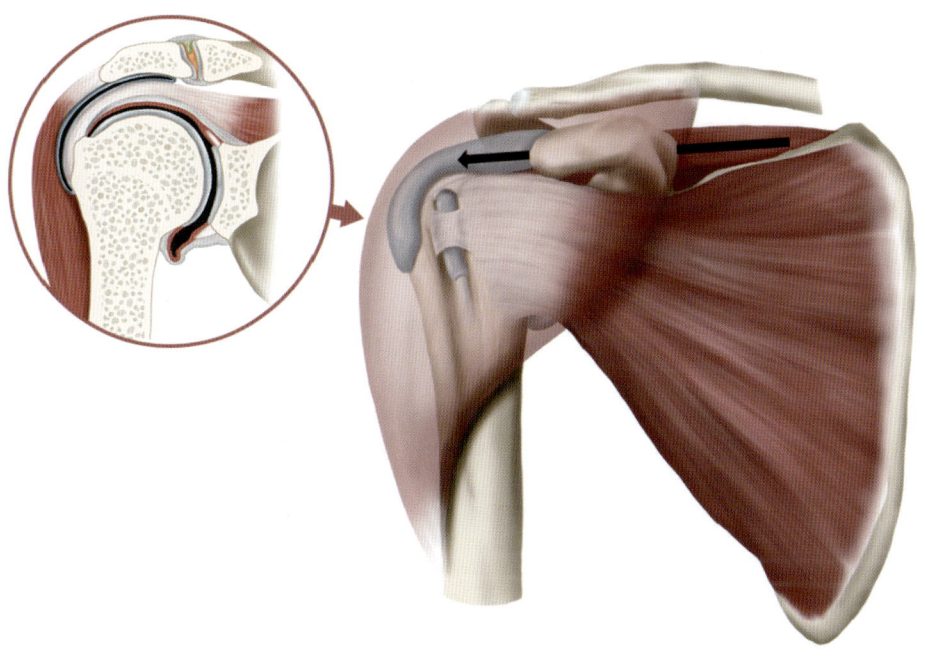

IV. Clinical Cases and Protocols

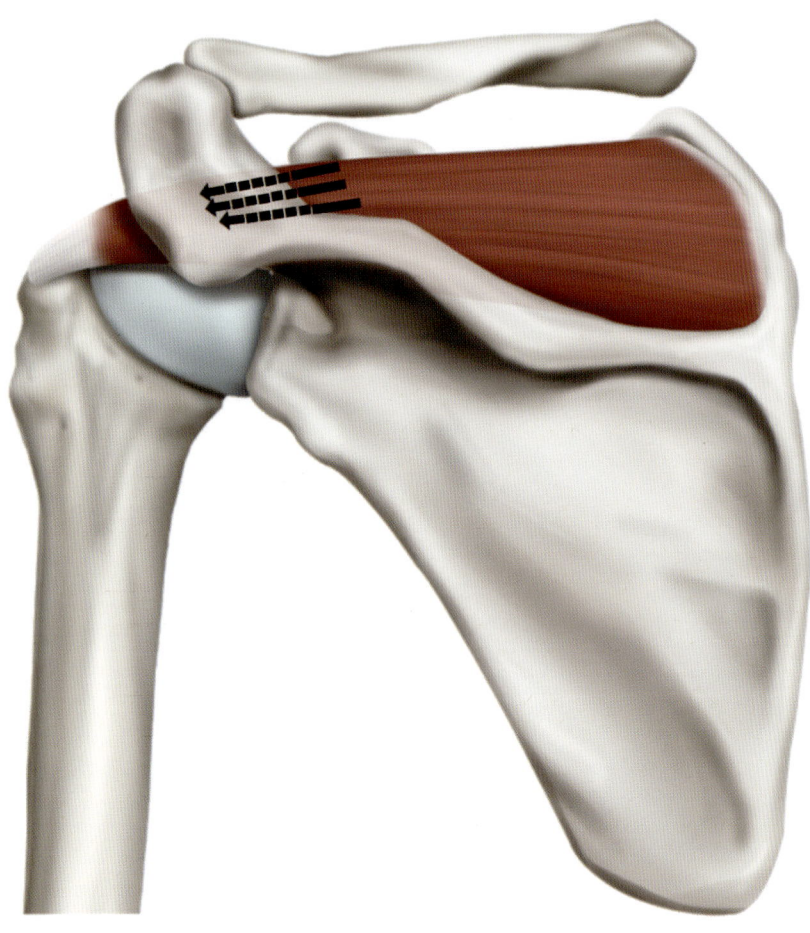

IV. Clinical Cases and Protocols

Shoulder Anatomy
(Lateral)

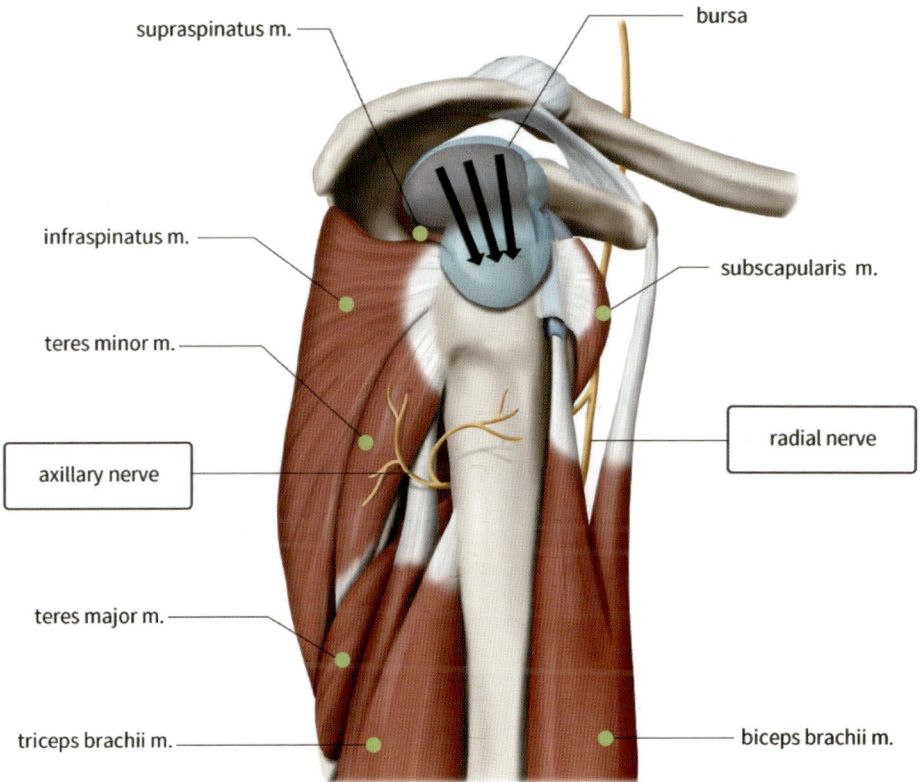

IV. Clinical Cases and Protocols

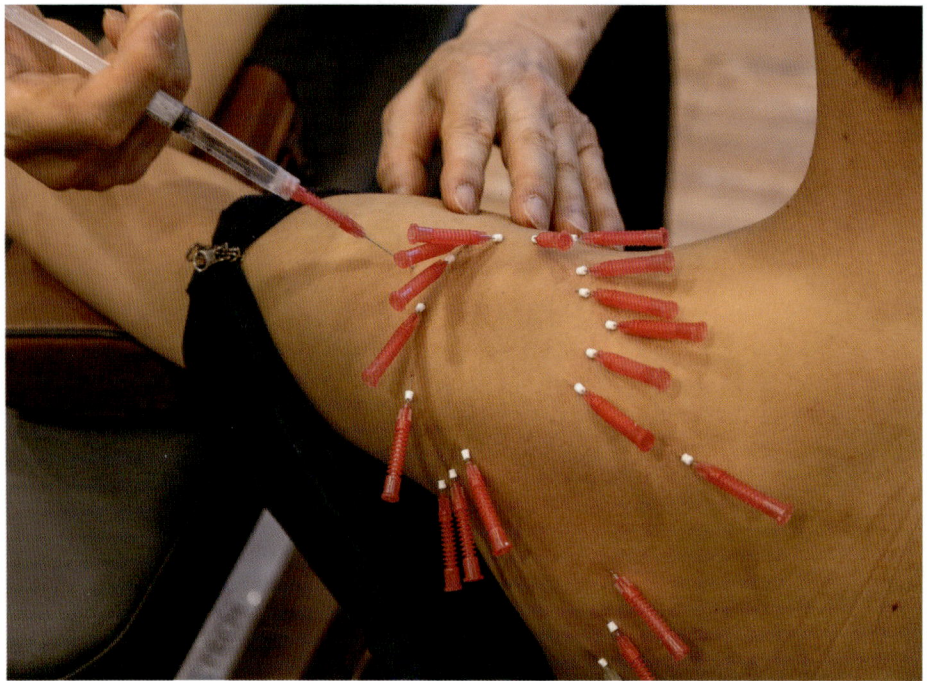

Insert threads transversely from the supraspinatus tendon toward the area over the subacromial bursa, and administer pharmacopuncture simultaneously.

For supraspinatus treatment, insert threads obliquely from the supraspinous fossa toward the subacromial bursa, performing pharmacopuncture at the same time.

IV. Clinical Cases and Protocols

Shoulder Anatomy
(Lateral)

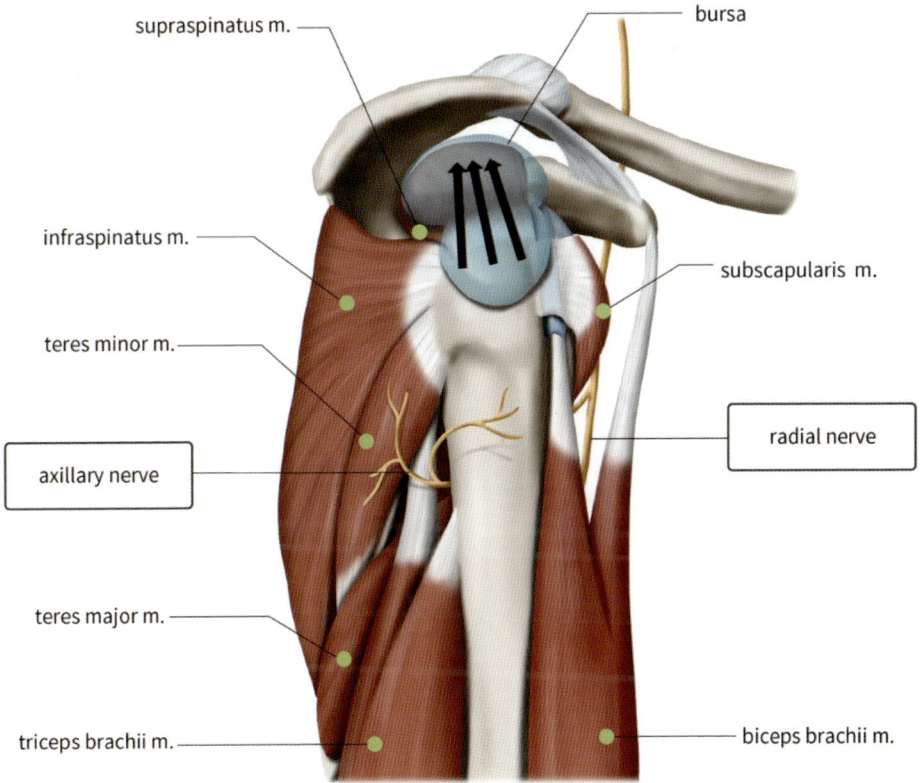

IV. Clinical Cases and Protocols

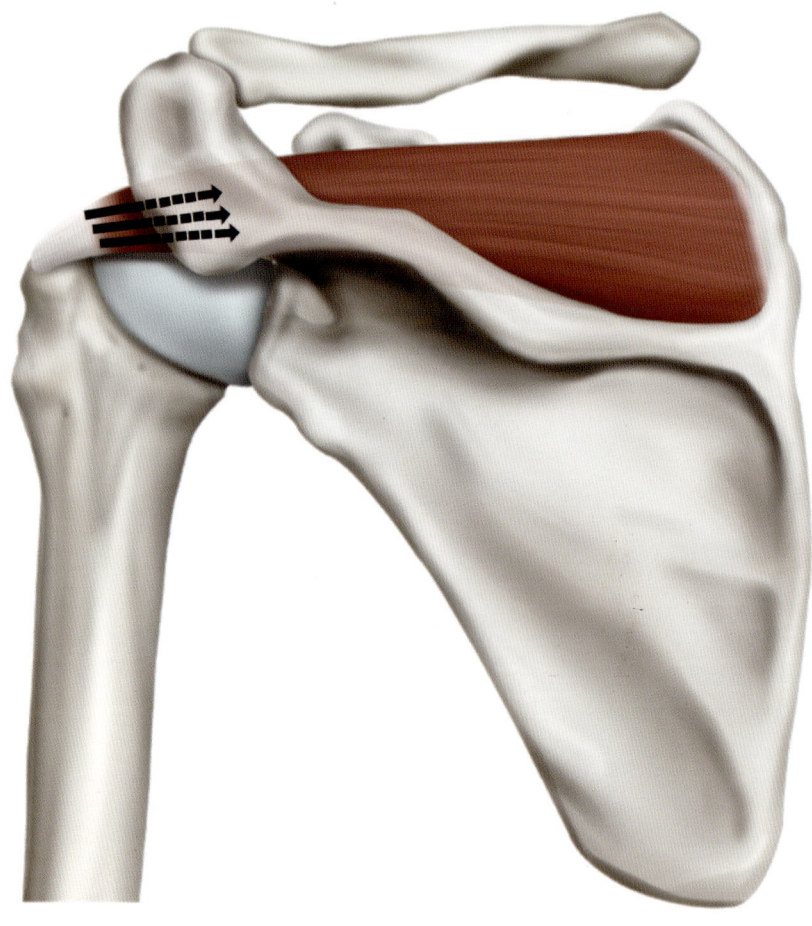

IV. Clinical Cases and Protocols

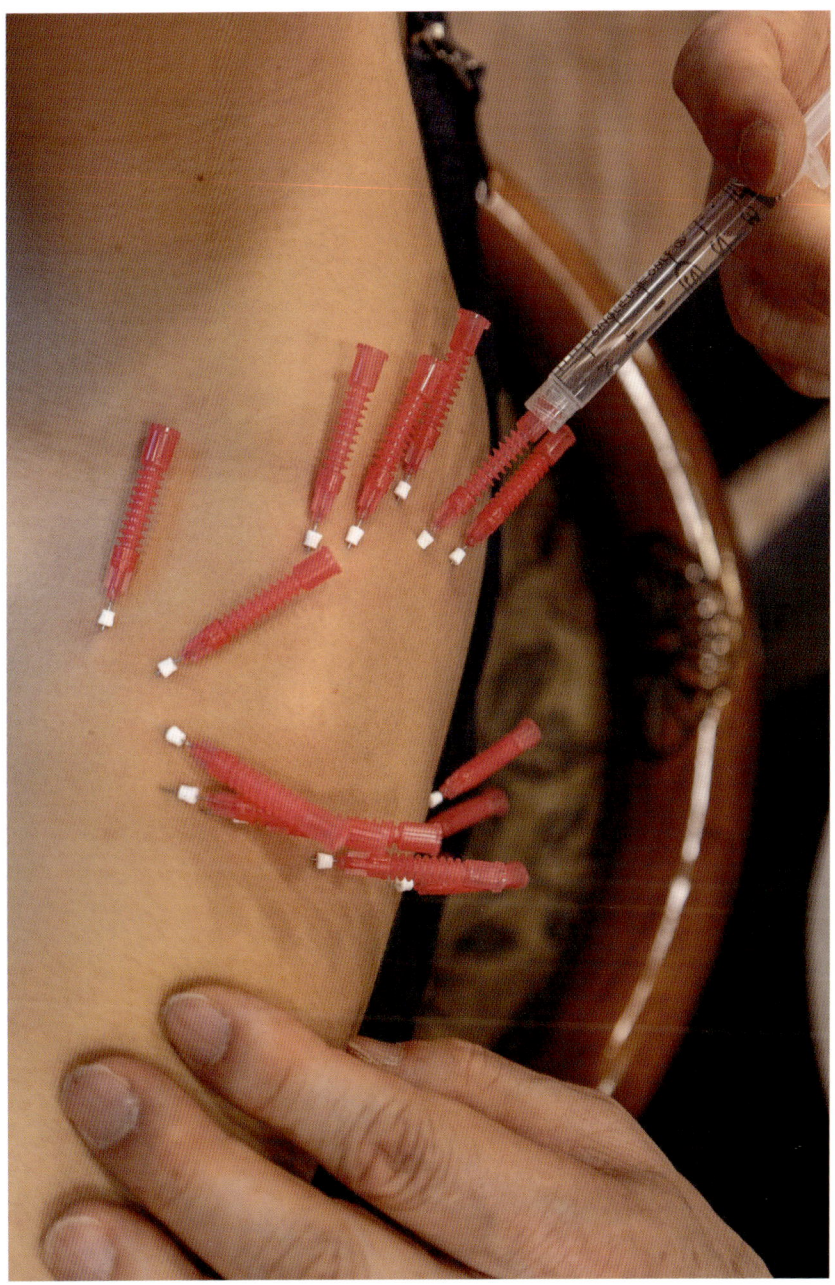

Insert threads transversely into the upper trapezius and supraspinatus muscles, and administer pharmacopuncture additionally at the same sites.

IV. Clinical Cases and Protocols

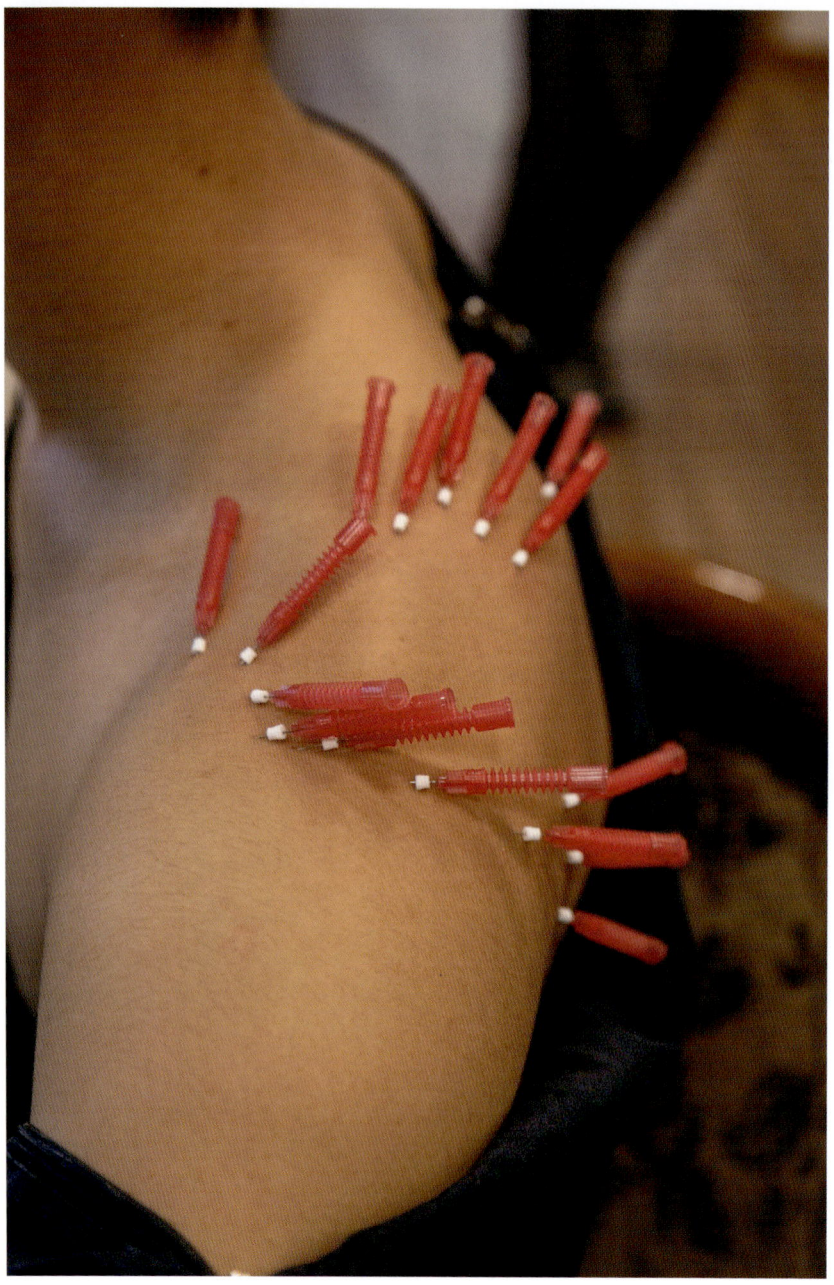

For the teres major muscle, insert the thread perpendicularly from the area near Jianjing(肩井,GB21) toward the lesser tubercle of the humerus.

IV. Clinical Cases and Protocols

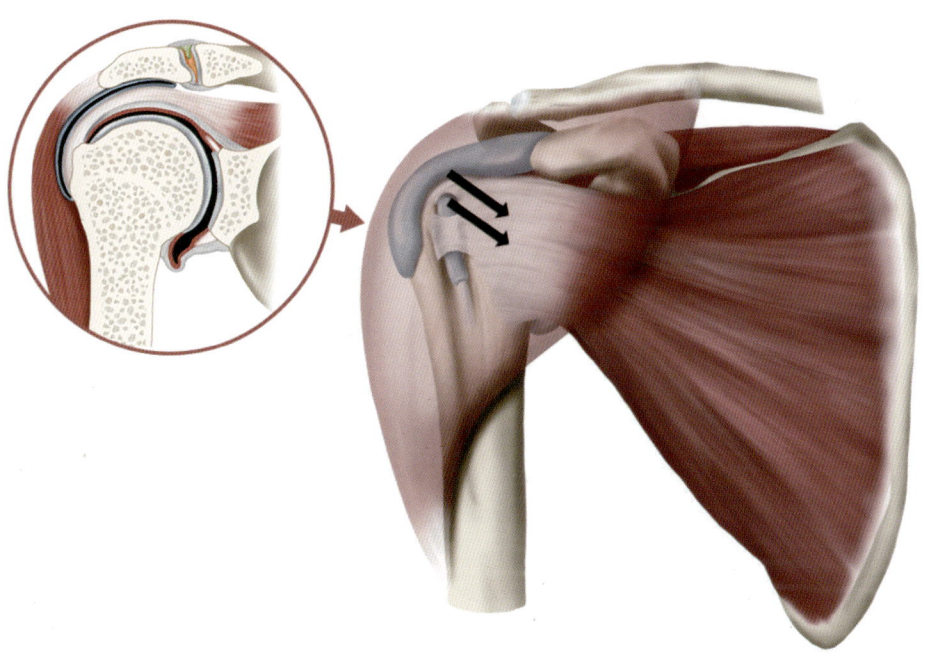

IV. Clinical Cases and Protocols

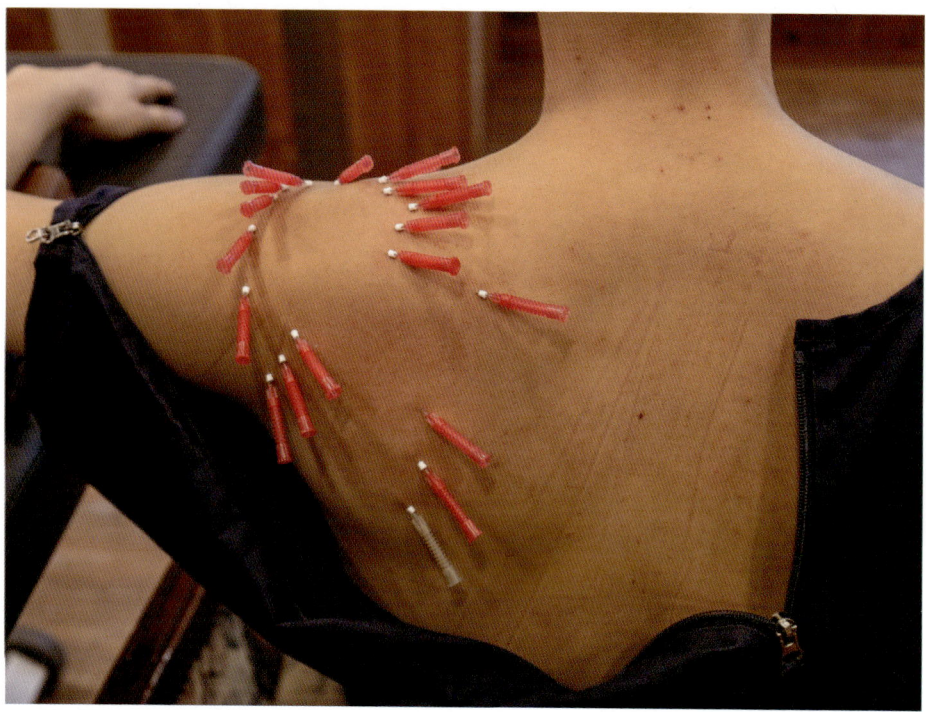

Insert threads obliquely into the infraspinatus and teres minor muscles, directing the insertion toward the humeral head.

IV. Clinical Cases and Protocols

Shoulder Anatomy

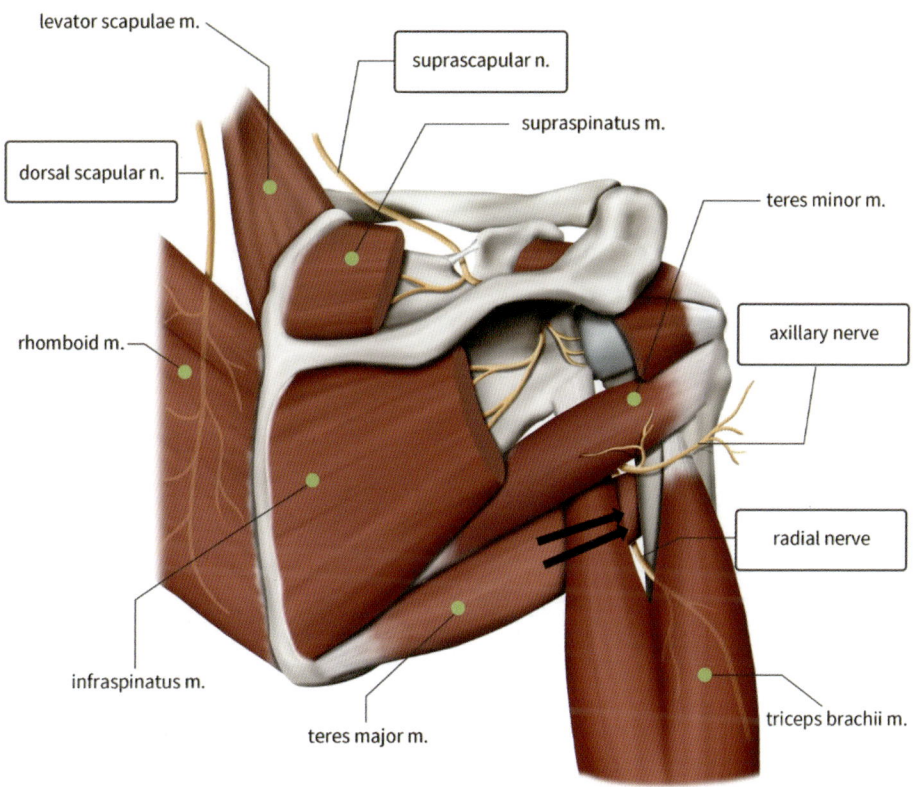

IV. Clinical Cases and Protocols

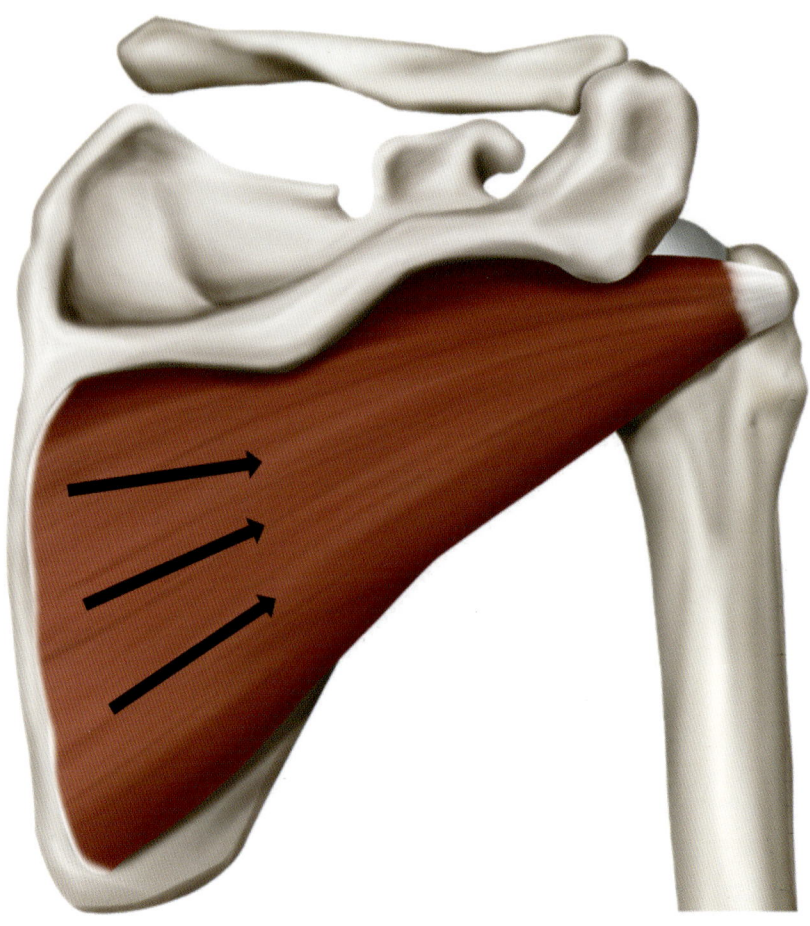

IV. Clinical Cases and Protocols

6. Elbow Joint

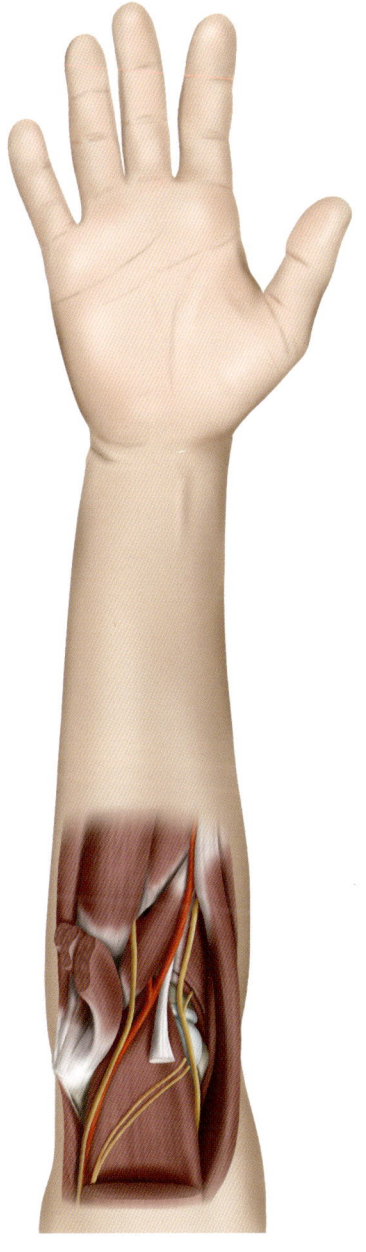
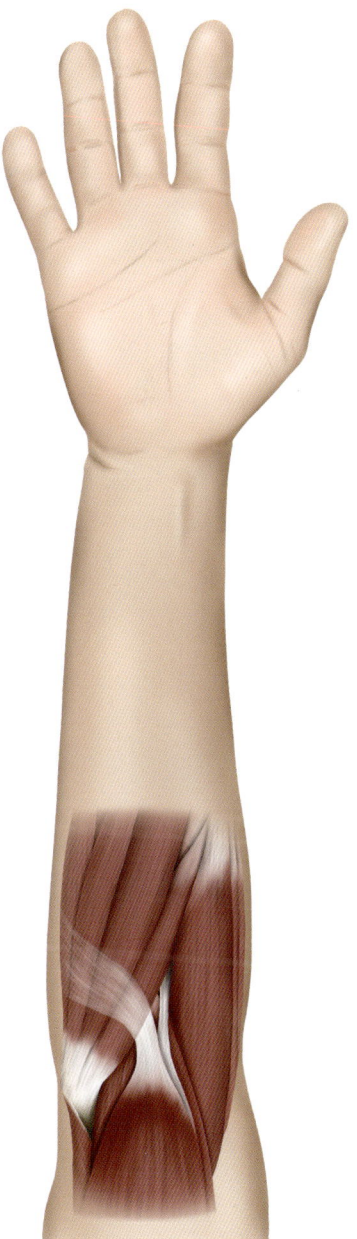

IV. Clinical Cases and Protocols

Lateral forearm muscles

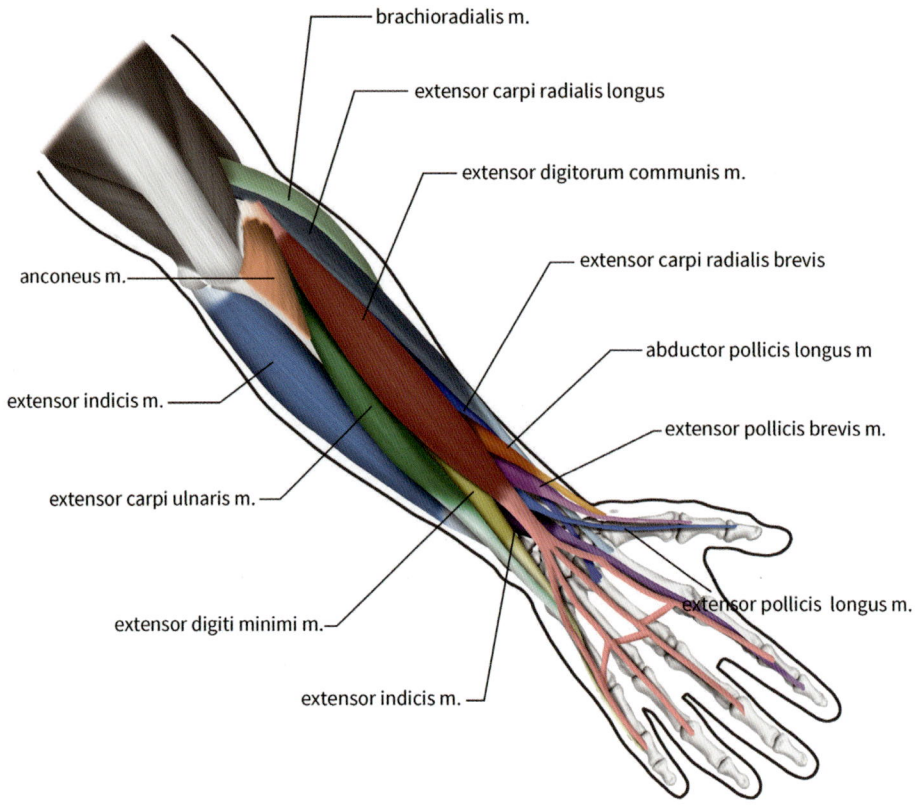

IV. Clinical Cases and Protocols

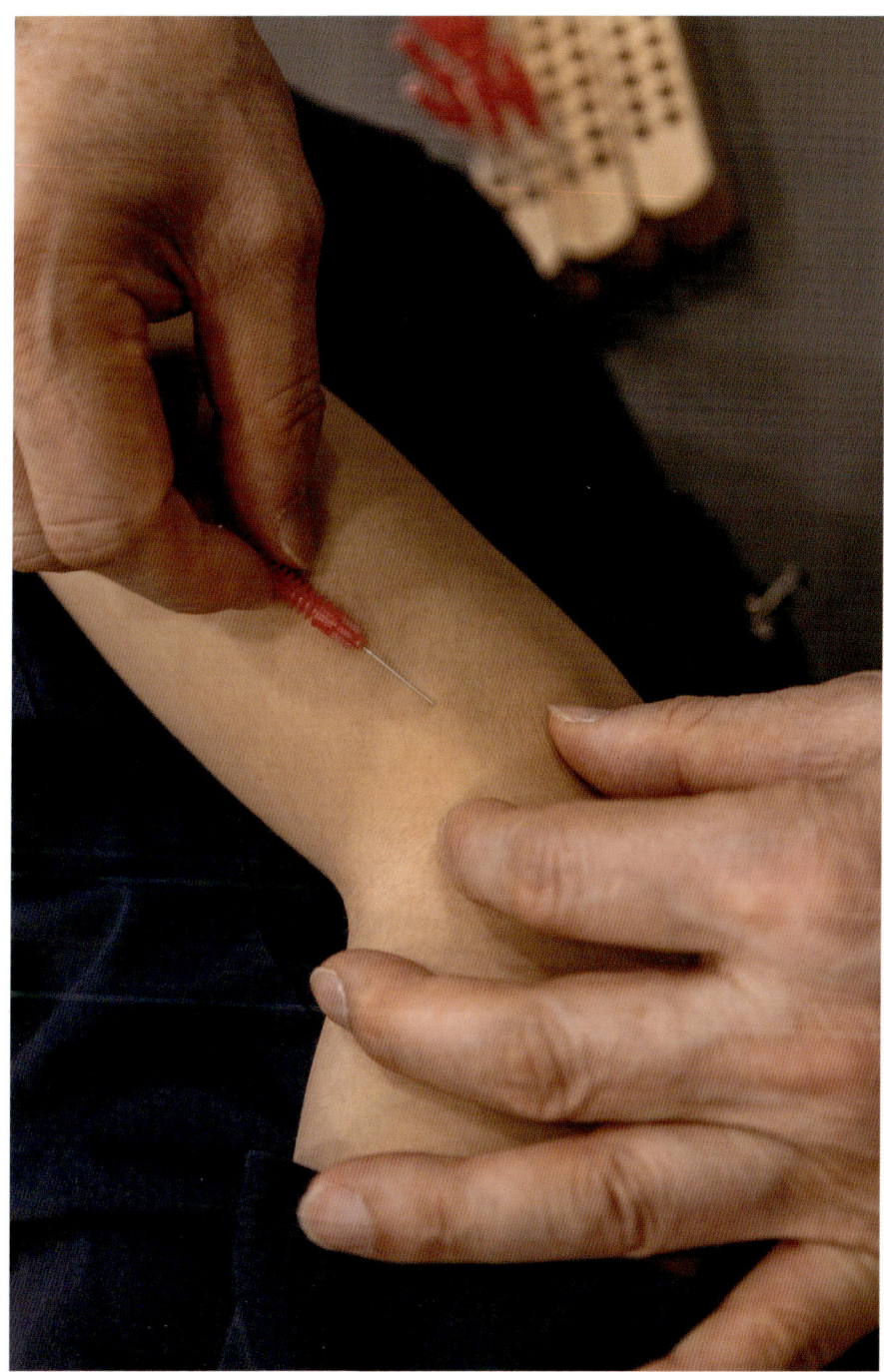

IV. Clinical Cases and Protocols

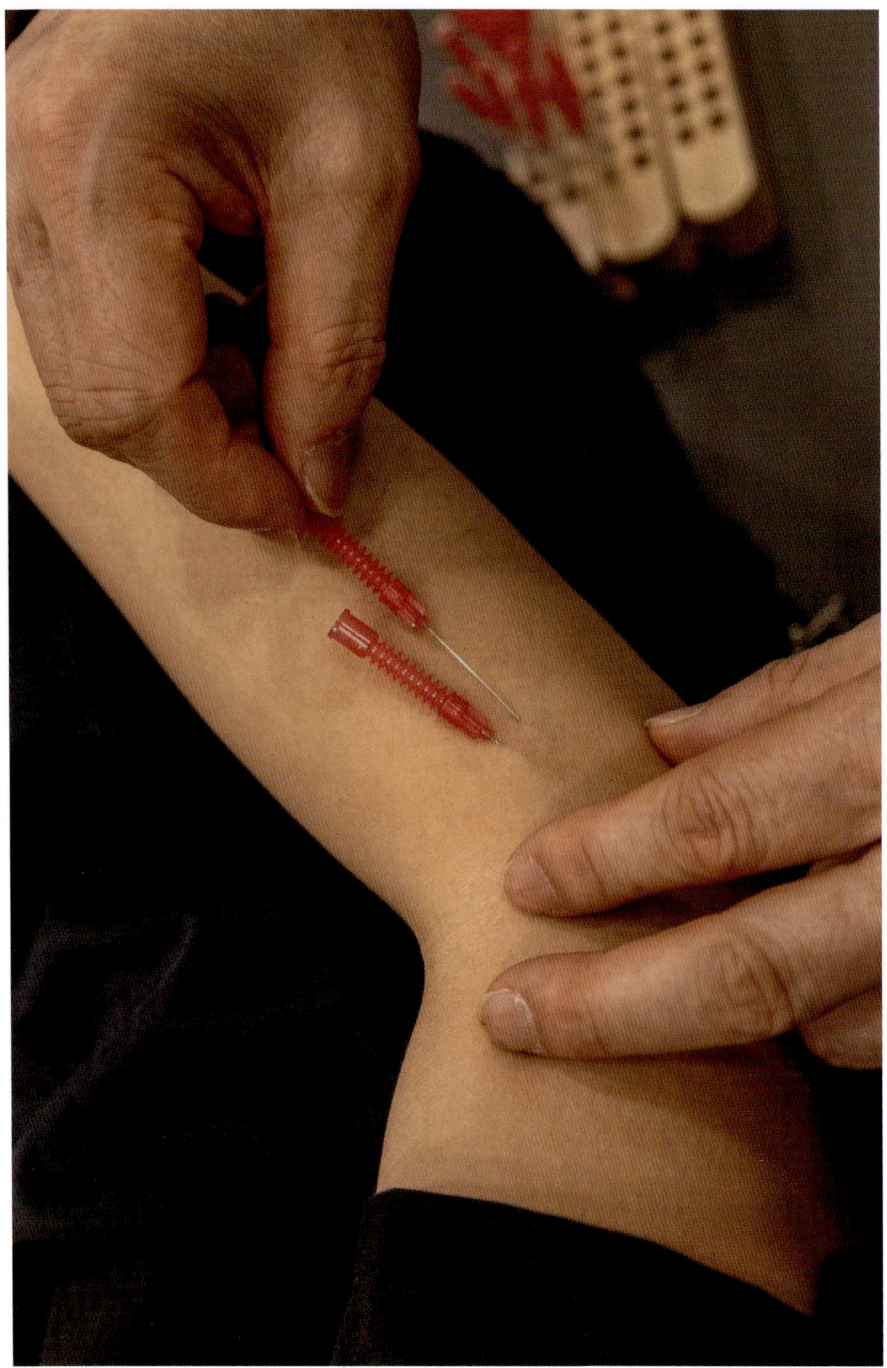

IV. Clinical Cases and Protocols

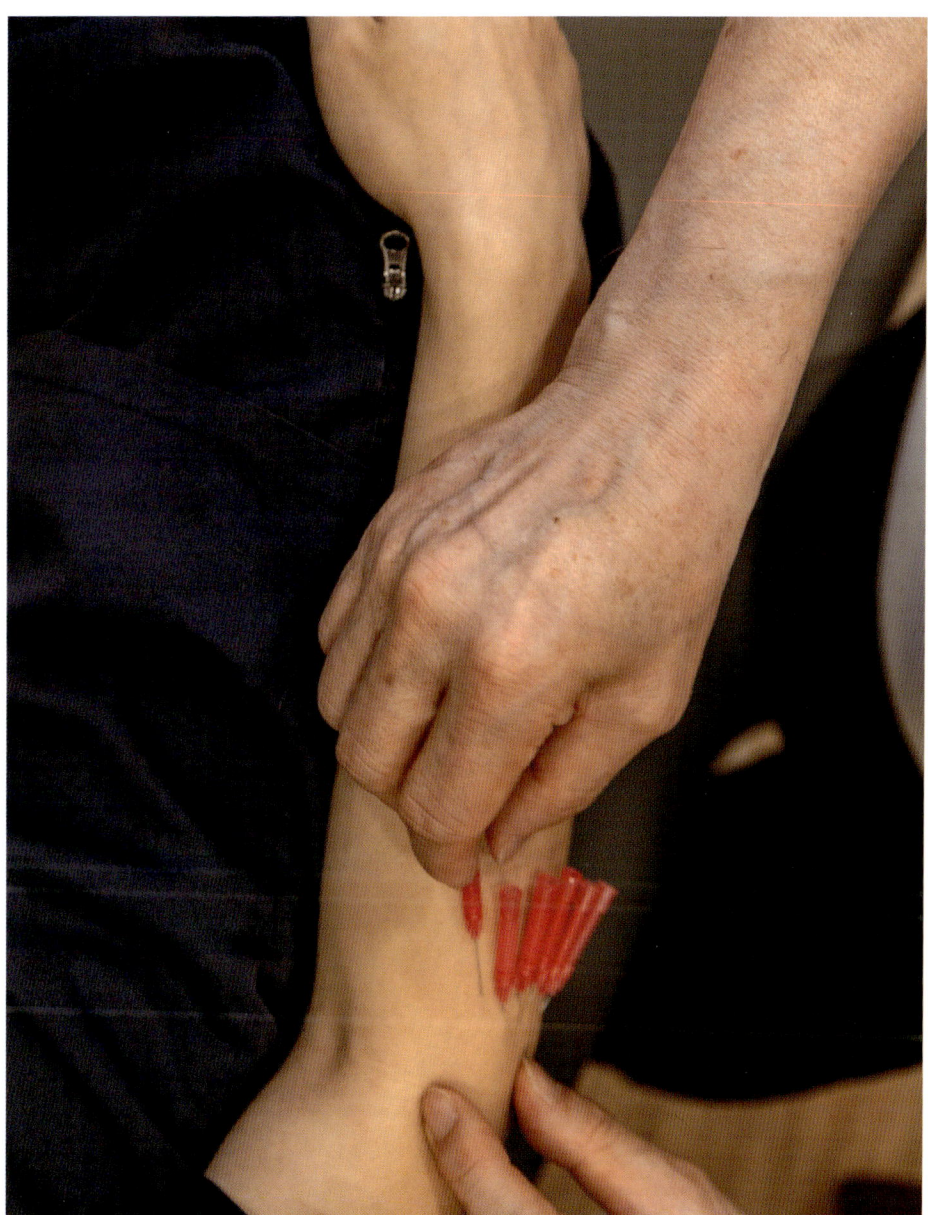

In cases of lateral epicondylitis (tennis elbow), assess for dysfunction in the muscles attaching to the lateral epicondyle of the humerus—including the extensor digitorum, extensor carpi radialis brevis, extensor carpi ulnaris, extensor digiti minimi, and supinator. Insert threads transversely into the affected muscles accordingly.

IV. Clinical Cases and Protocols

Lateral forearm muscles

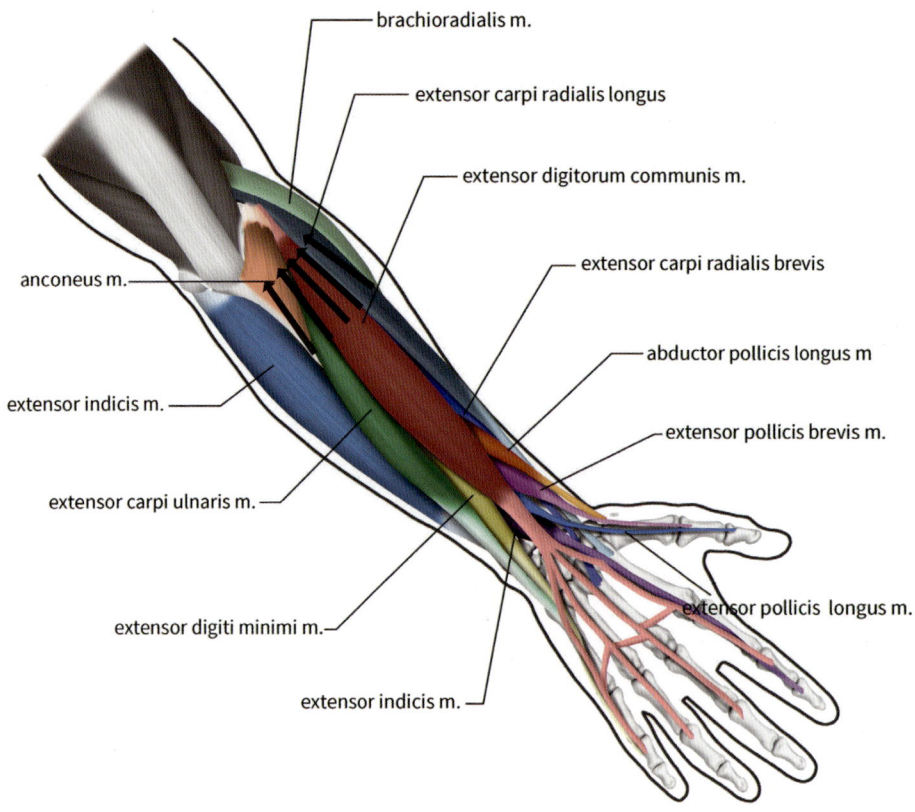

IV. Clinical Cases and Protocols

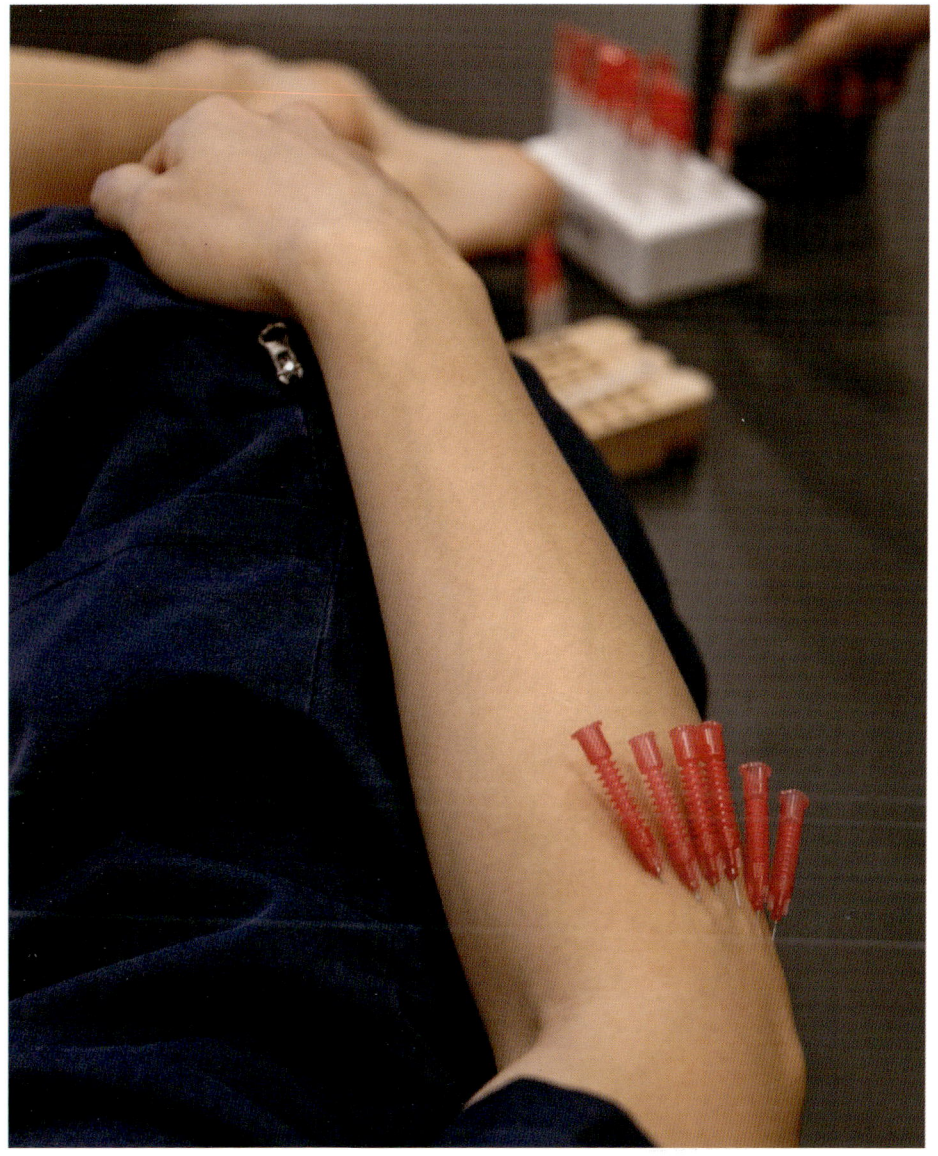

IV. Clinical Cases and Protocols

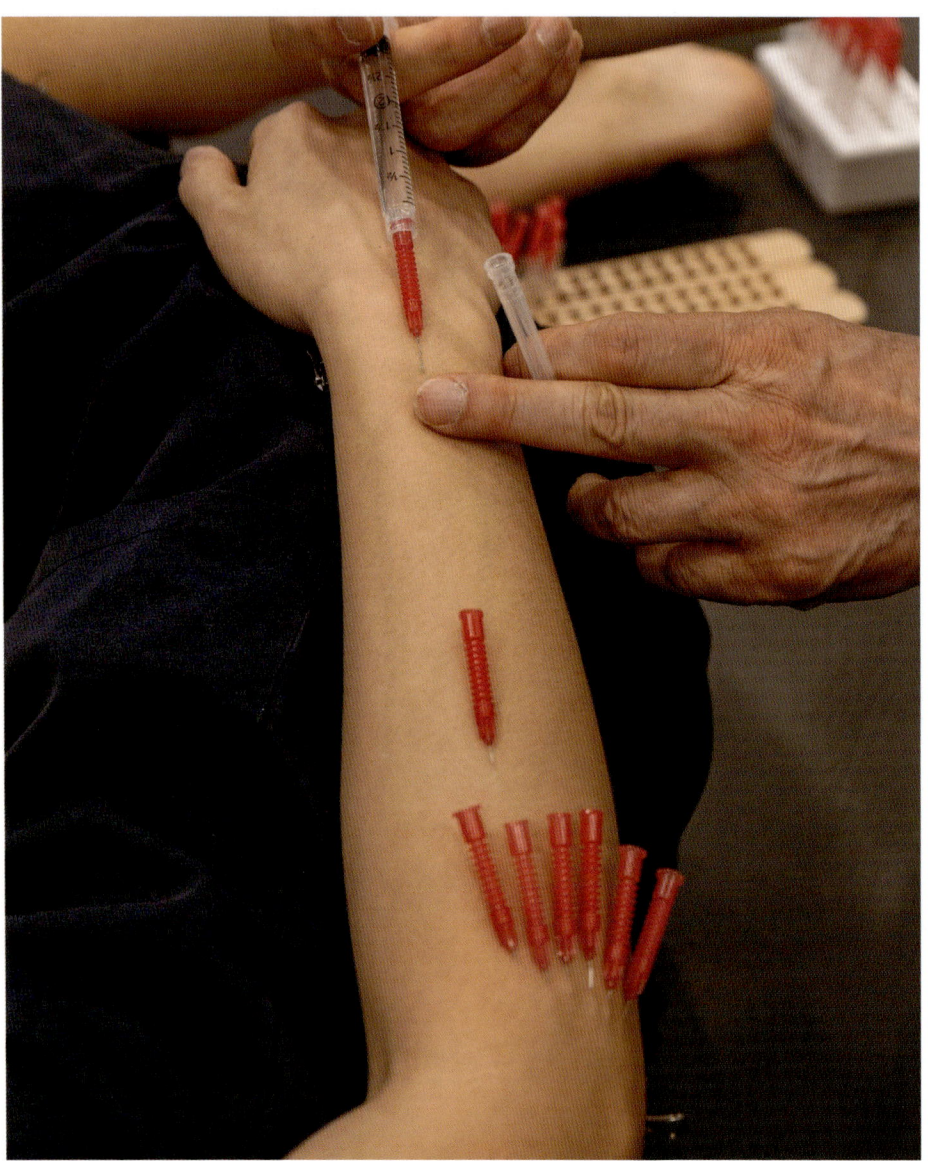

Identify tender points near Shousanli (手三里, LI10) and insert threads transversely. Also insert threads transversely around the wrist area—such as near Waiguan (外關, SJ5) or into nearby muscles—and administer pharmacopuncture at these sites.

Lateral forearm muscles

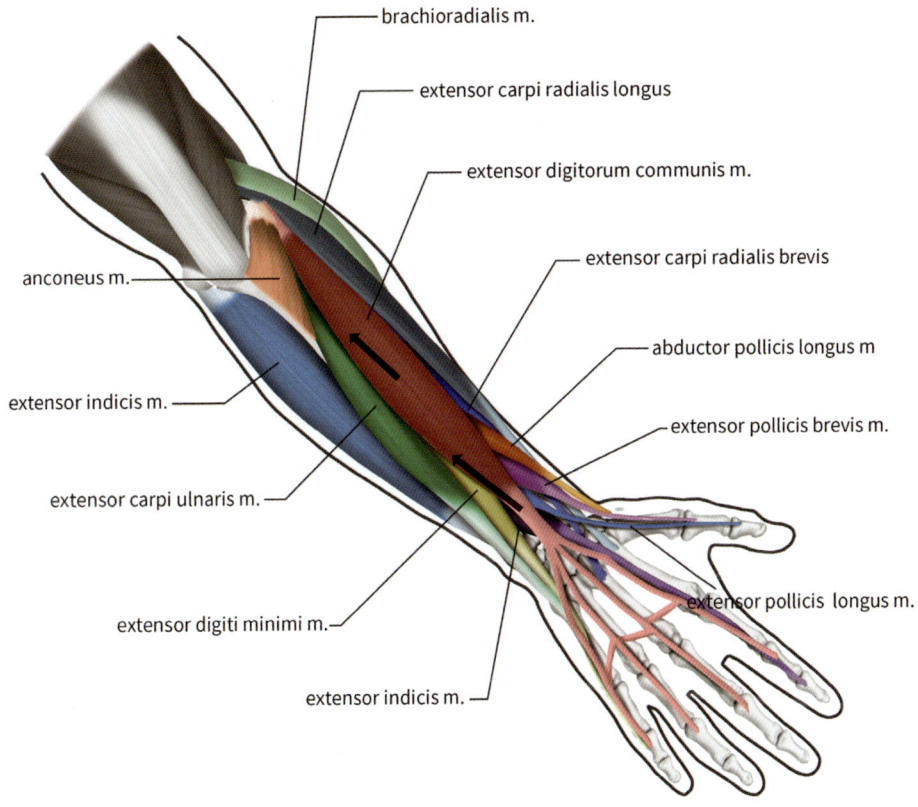

IV. Clinical Cases and Protocols

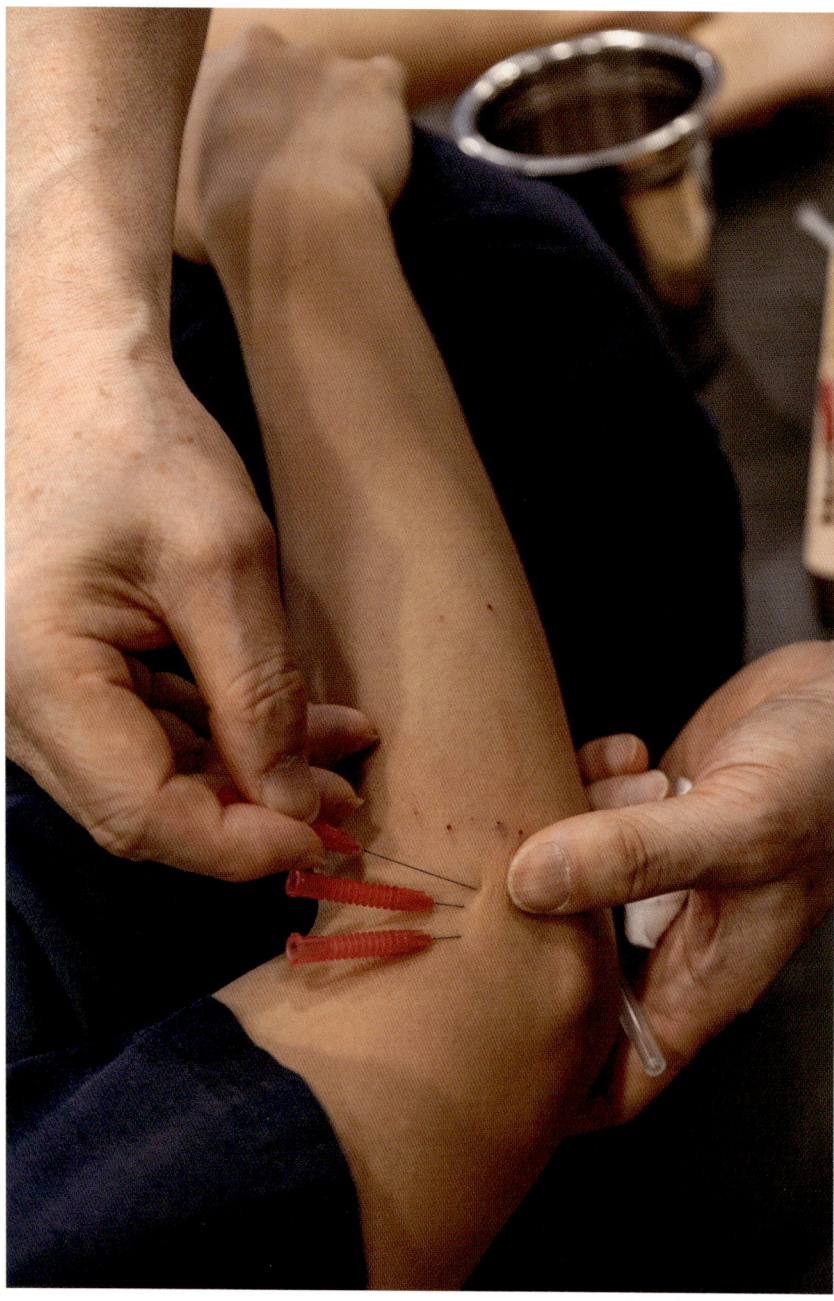

IV. Clinical Cases and Protocols

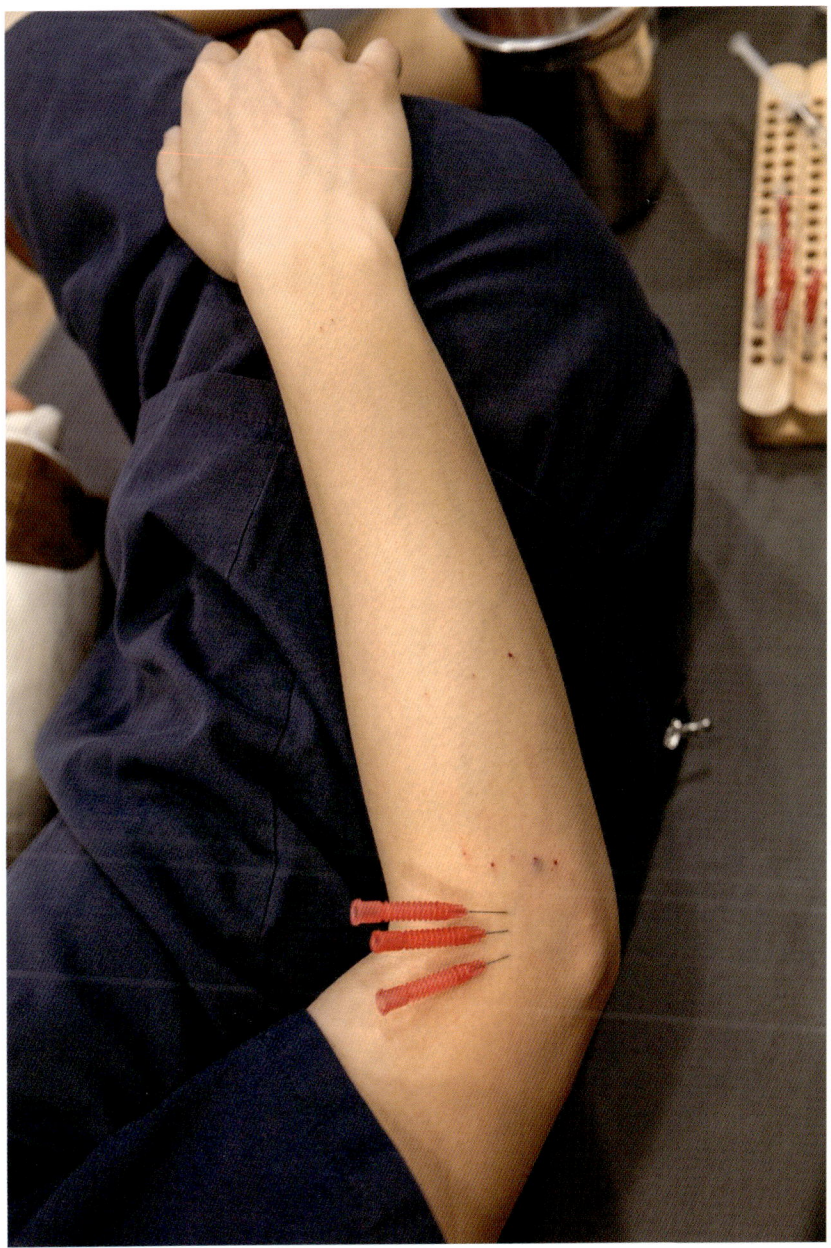

In cases of sprain involving the radial collateral ligament and annular ligament, perform thread embedding and pharmacopuncture simultaneously near the Quchi (曲池, LI11) point, directing the insertion toward the injured ligaments.

IV. Clinical Cases and Protocols

Lateral forearm muscles

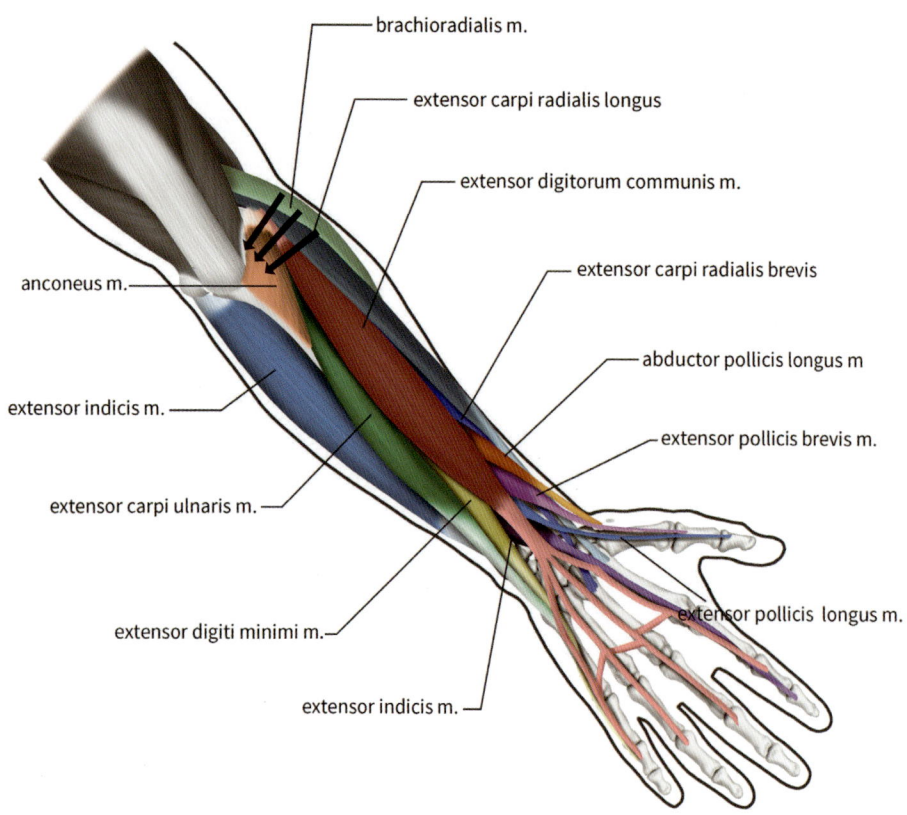

IV. Clinical Cases and Protocols

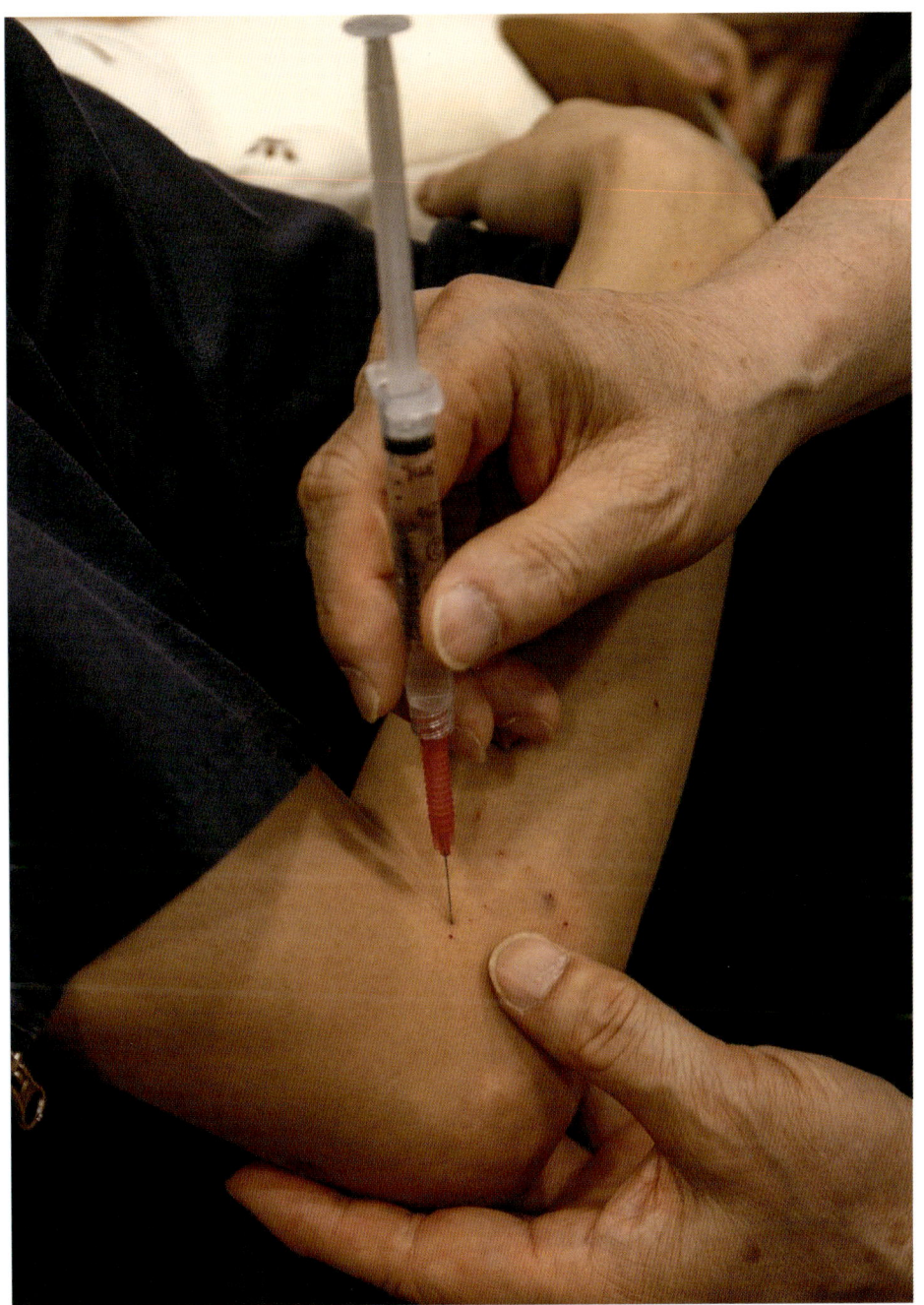

IV. Clinical Cases and Protocols

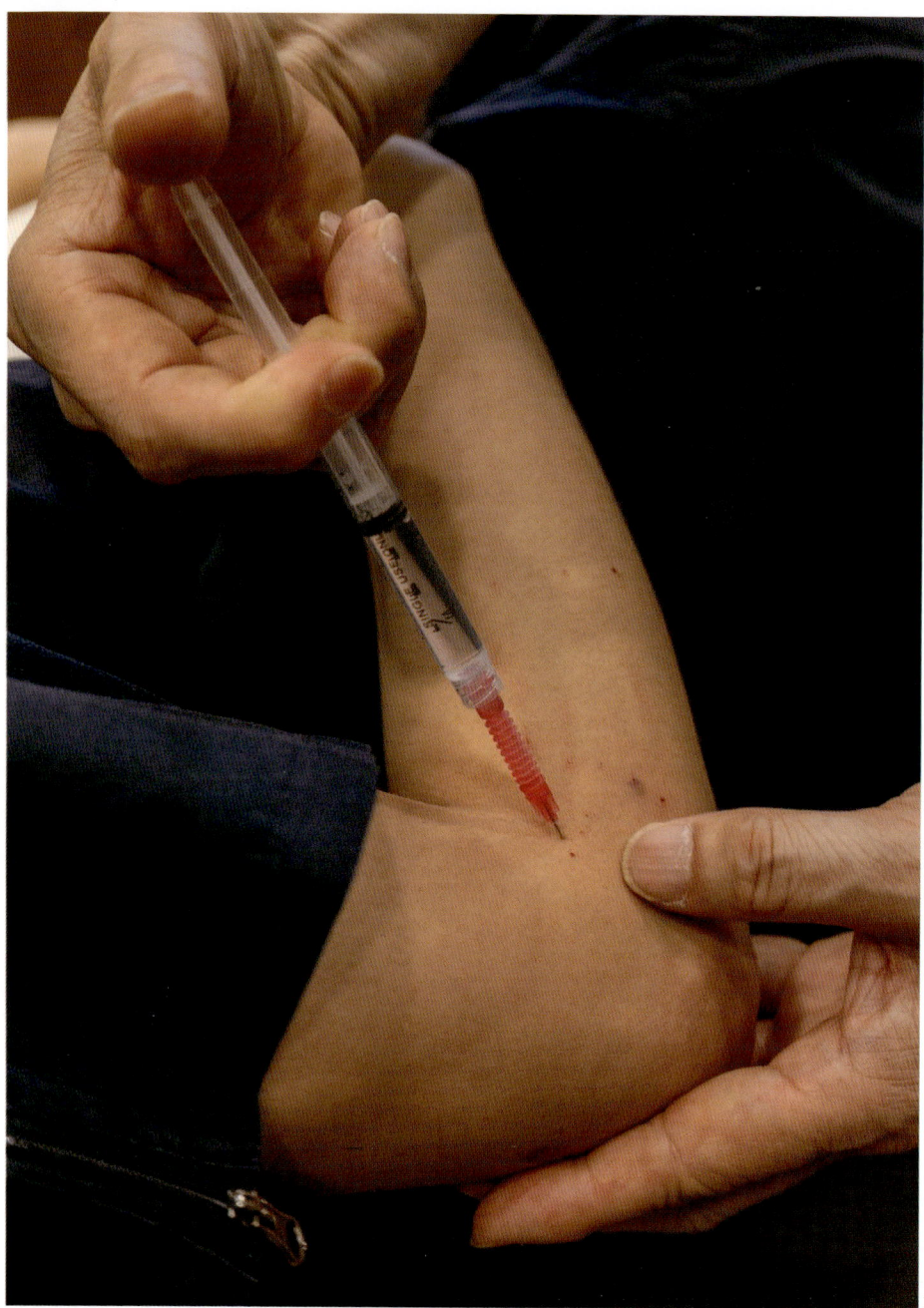

Combining transverse thread embedding with pharmacopuncture enhances therapeutic effectiveness.

IV. Clinical Cases and Protocols

Medial forearm muscles

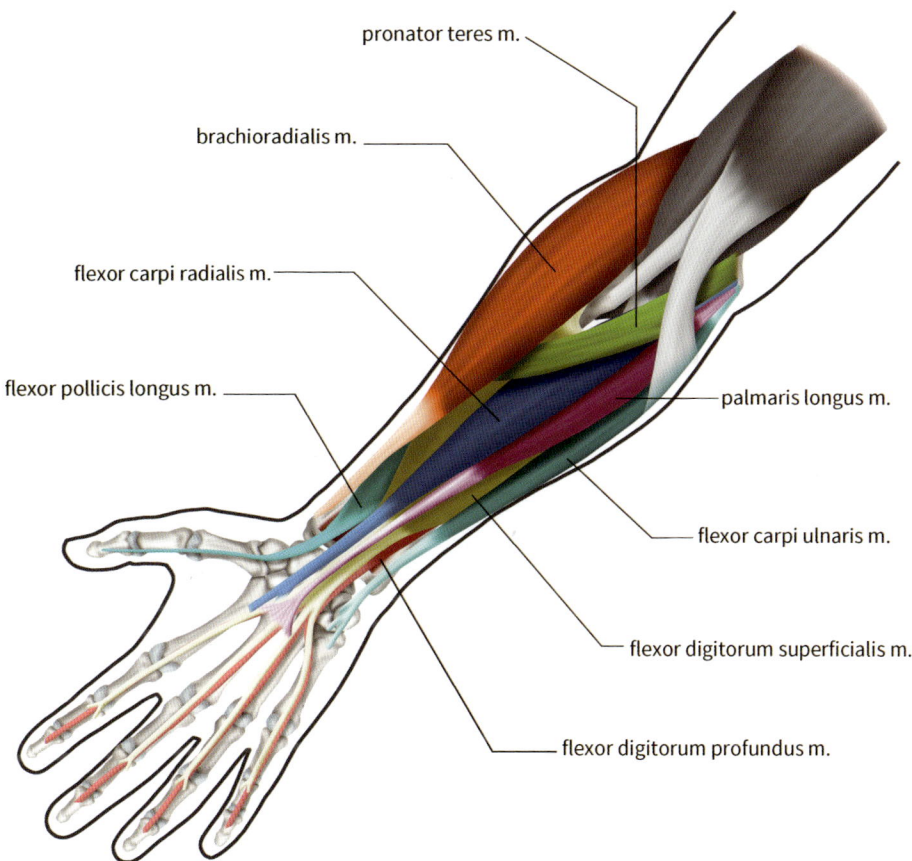

IV. Clinical Cases and Protocols

Cubital tunnel

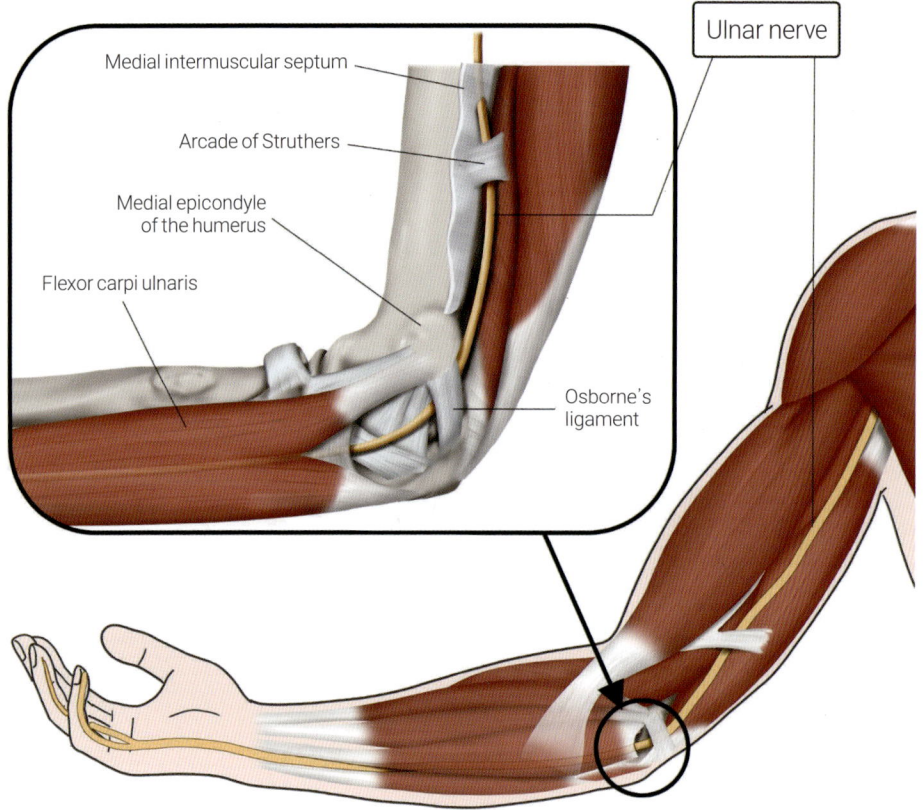

IV. Clinical Cases and Protocols

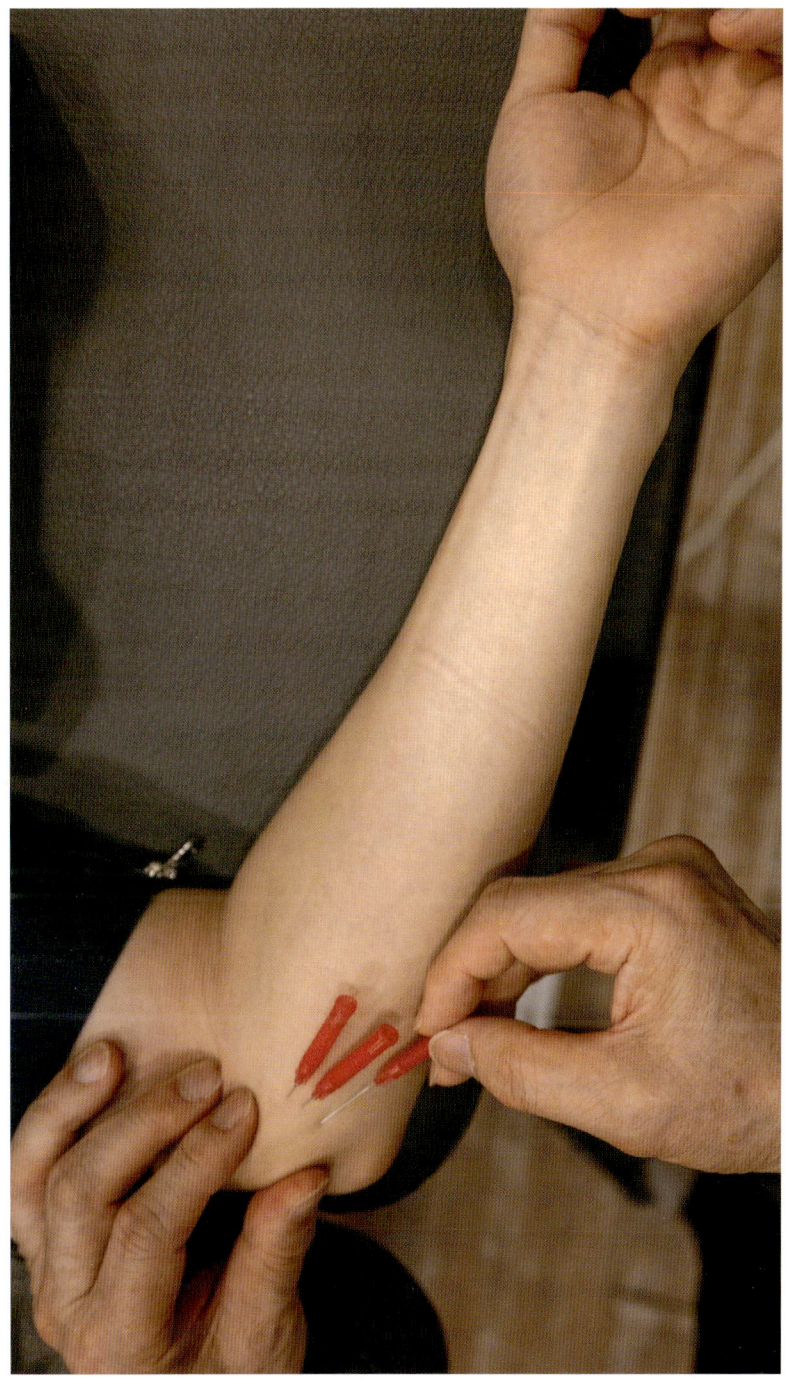

IV. Clinical Cases and Protocols

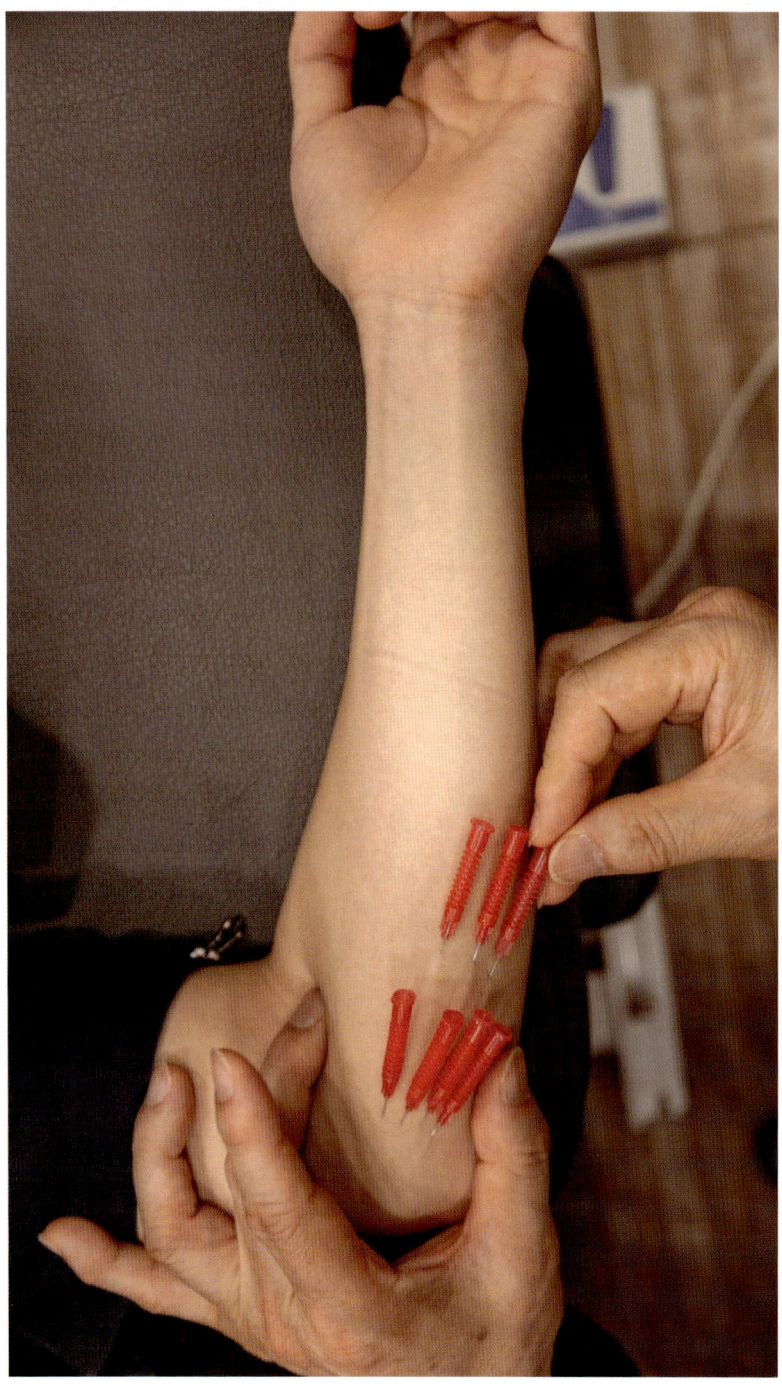

IV. Clinical Cases and Protocols

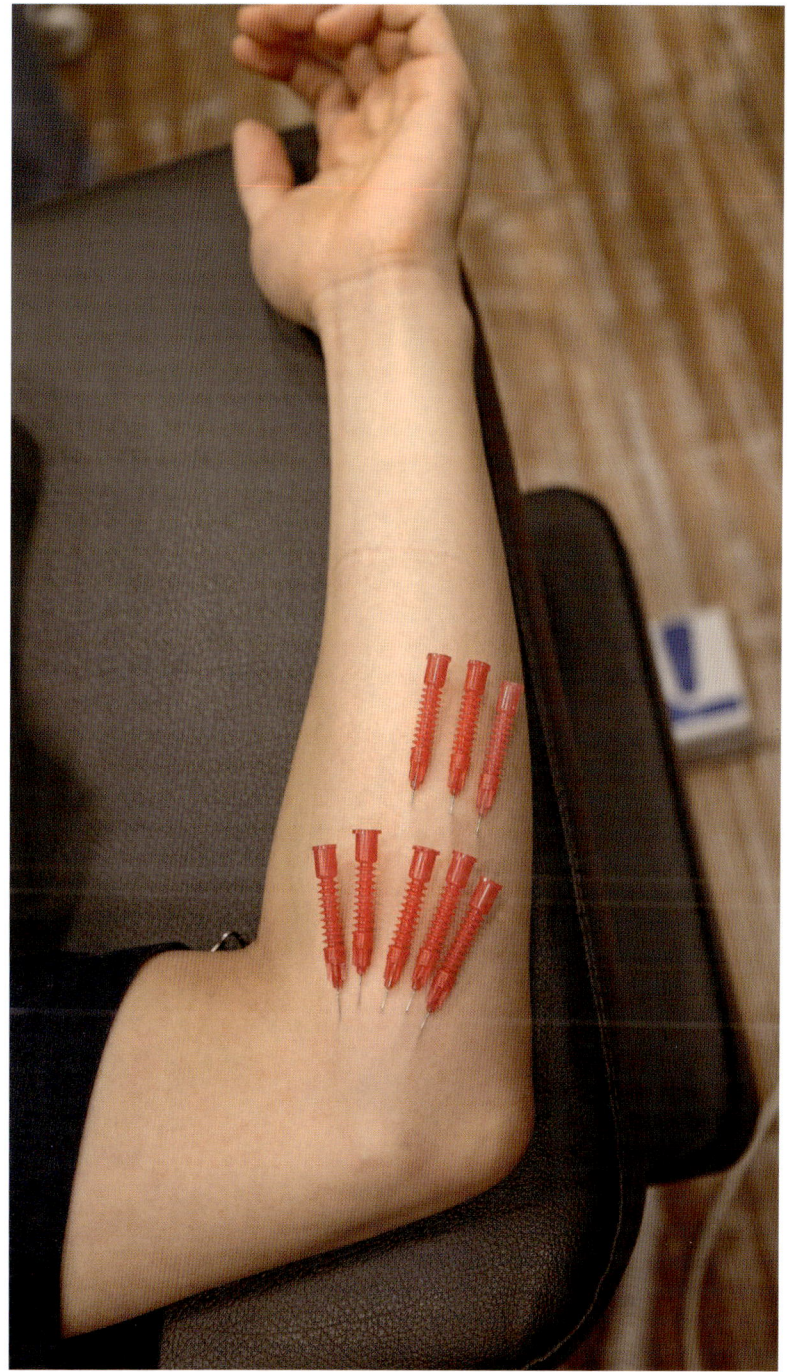

IV. Clinical Cases and Protocols

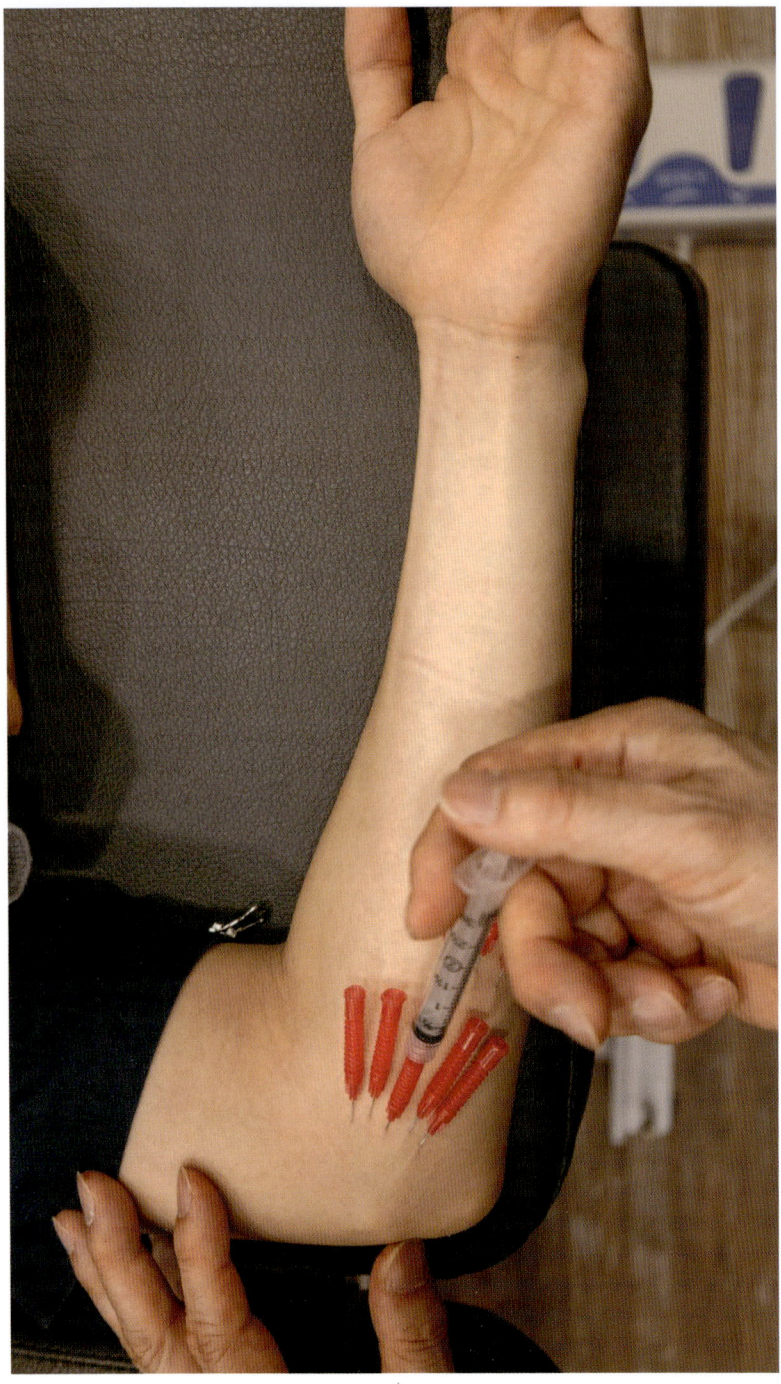

IV. Clinical Cases and Protocols

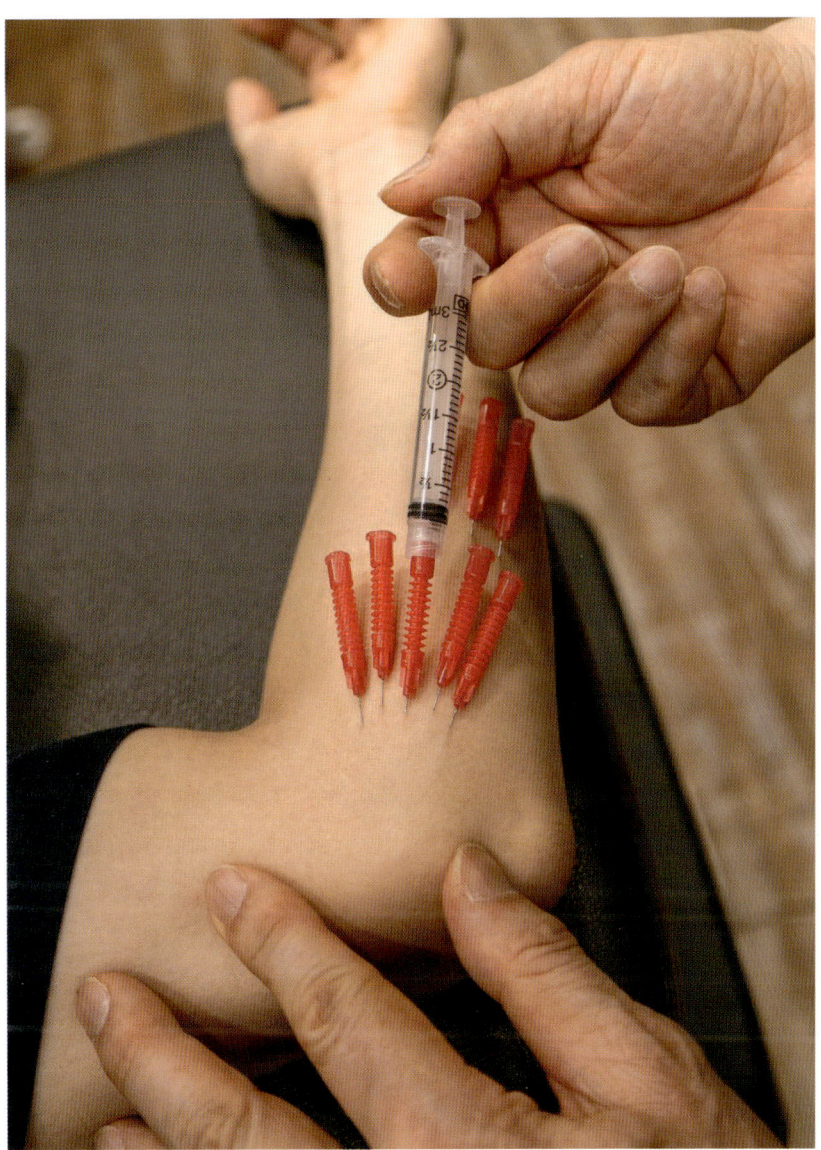

Assess for dysfunction in the muscles attached to the medial epicondyle of the humerus—including the pronator teres, flexor carpi radialis, palmaris longus, flexor carpi ulnaris, and flexor digitorum superficialis—and insert threads transversely into the affected muscles.

Thread embedding and pharmacopuncture may also be applied near Shaohai (小海, HT3) for enhanced effect.

IV. Clinical Cases and Protocols

Medial forearm muscles

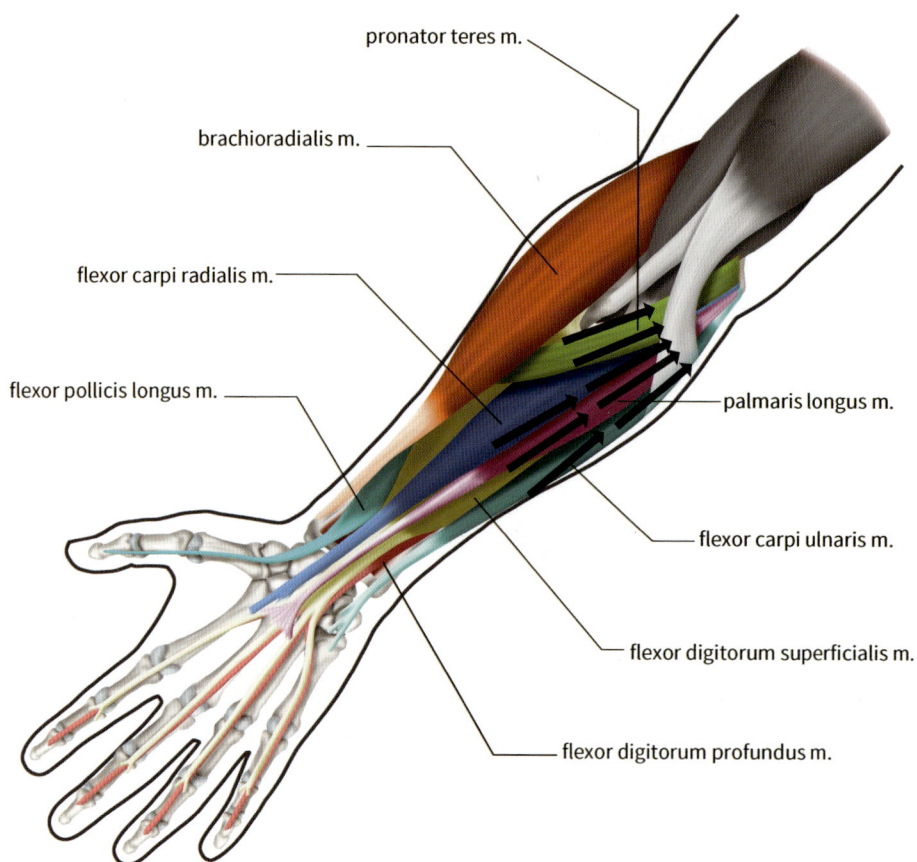

IV. Clinical Cases and Protocols

7. Wrist Joint

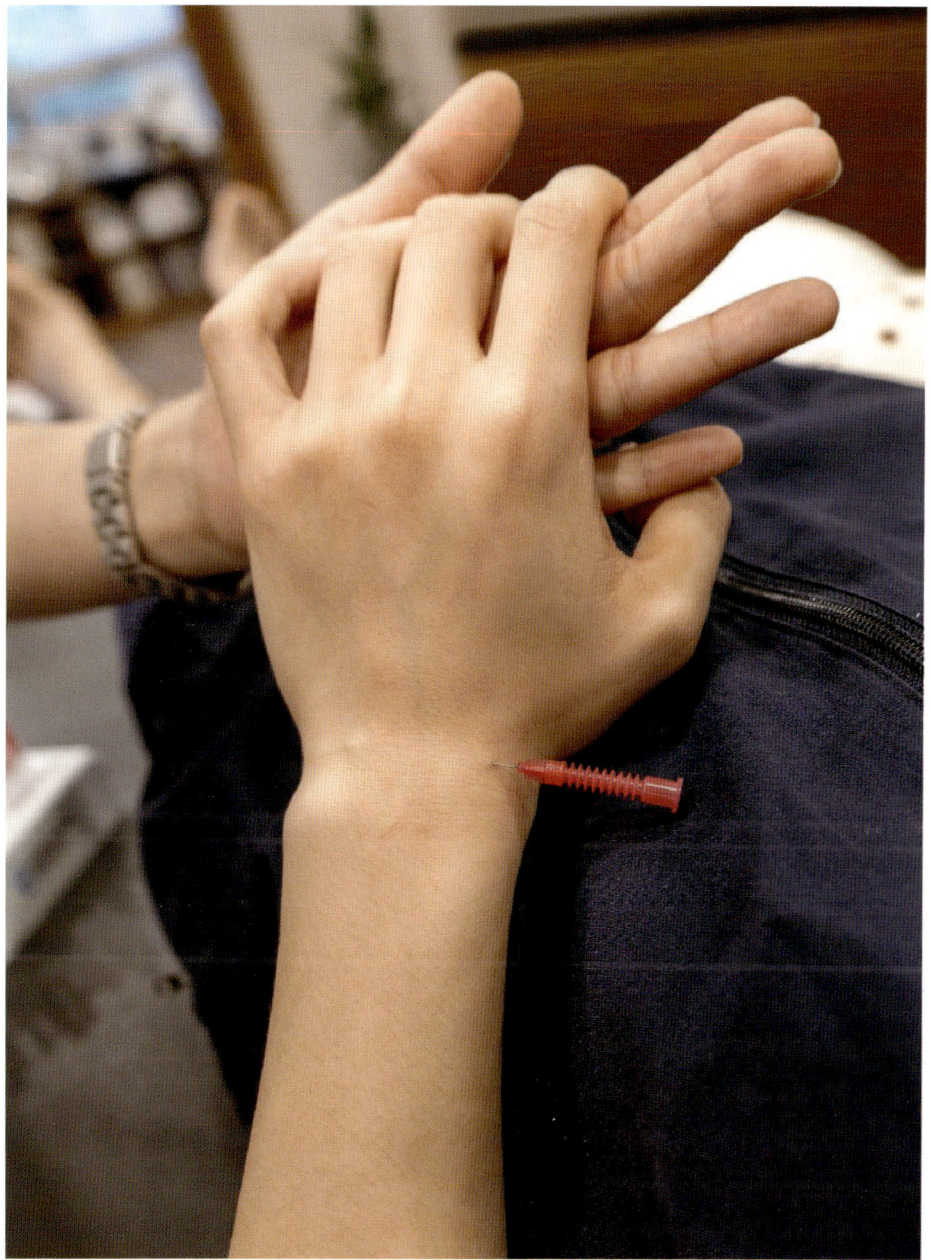

IV. Clinical Cases and Protocols

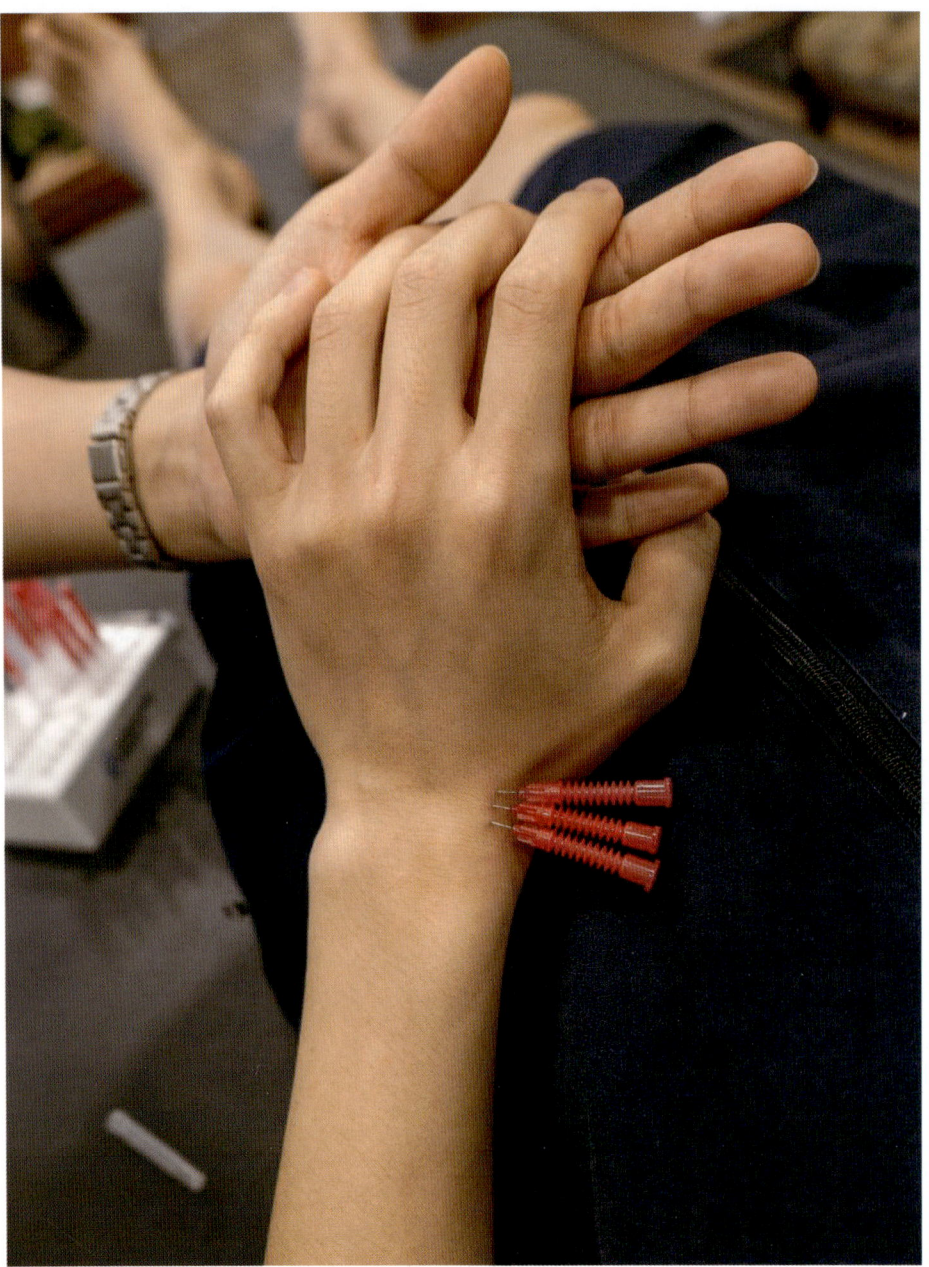

Insert threads transversely over the extensor retinaculum.

IV. Clinical Cases and Protocols

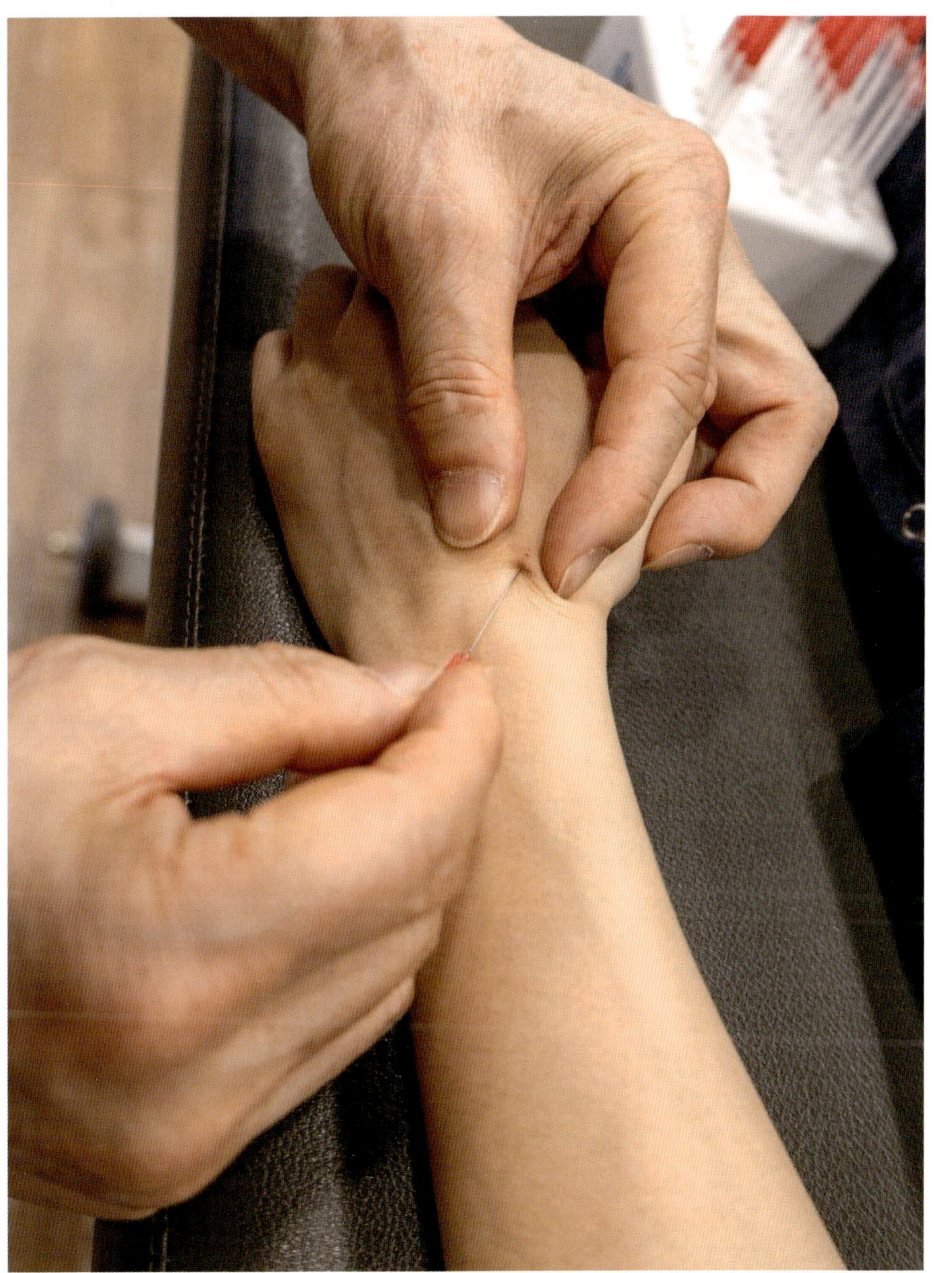

IV. Clinical Cases and Protocols

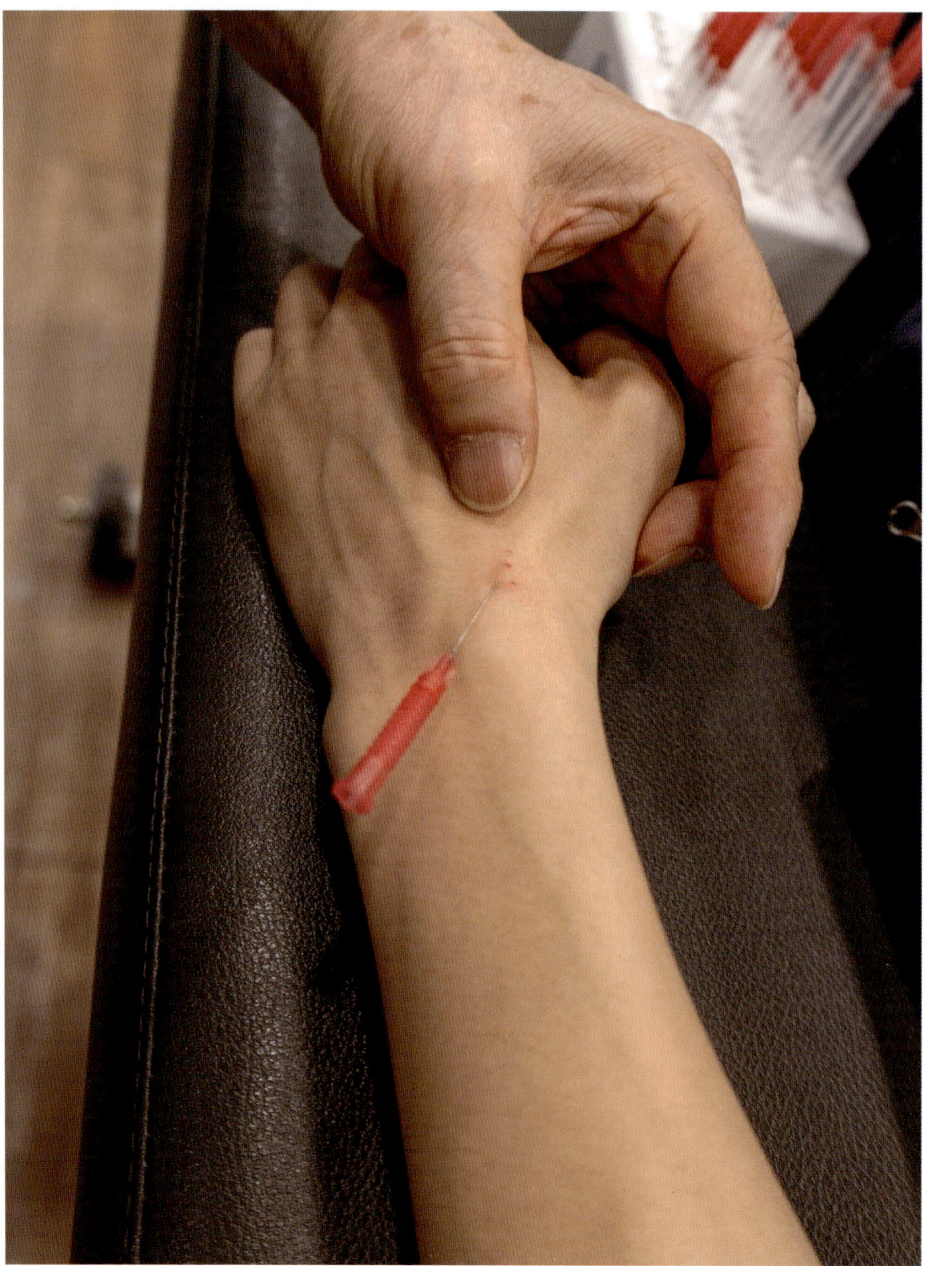

If there is dysfunction in the extensor pollicis longus, thread embedding and pharmacopuncture can be performed simultaneously along the direction of the tendon, targeting the tendon sheath.

IV. Clinical Cases and Protocols

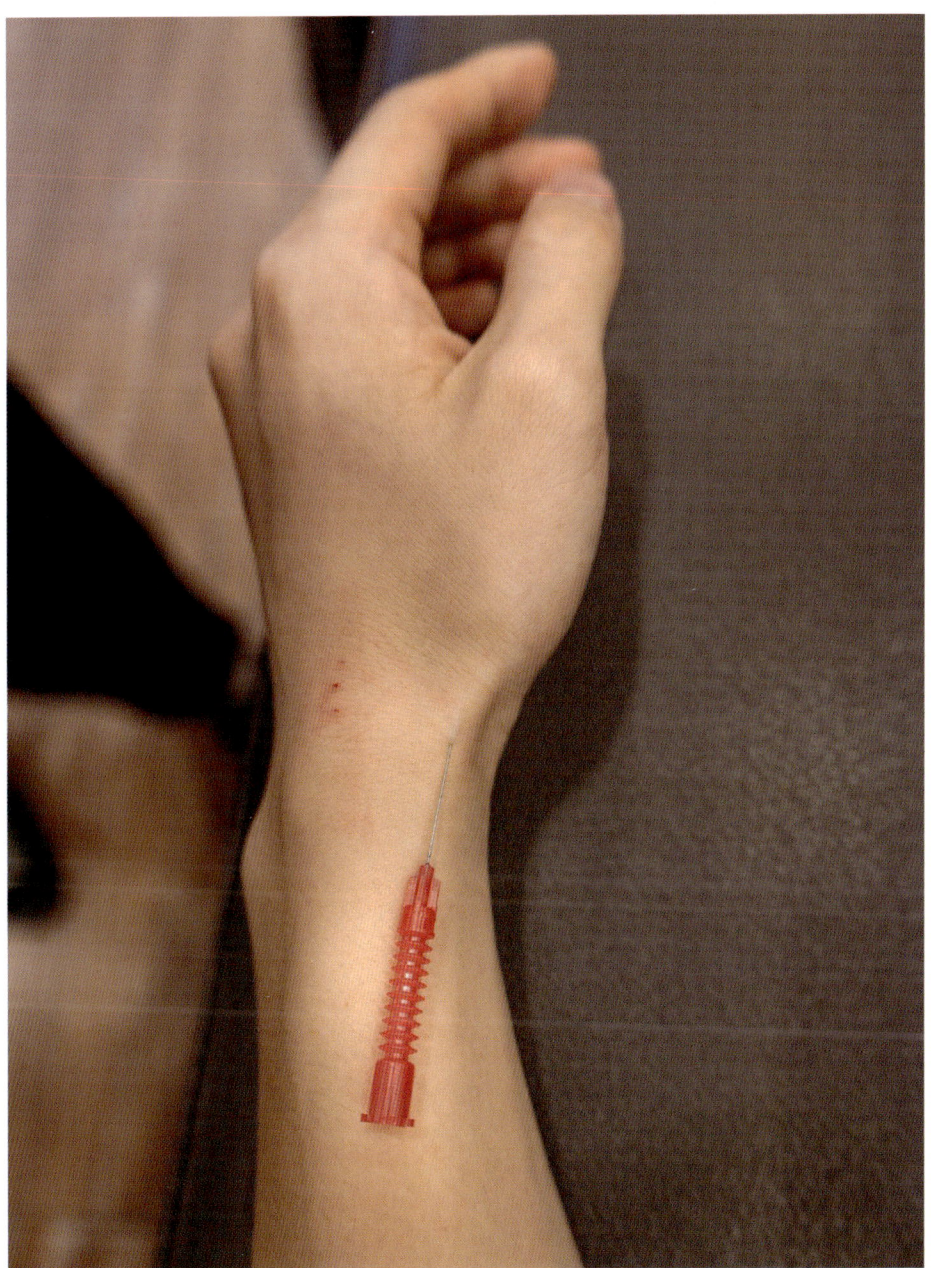

For the extensor pollicis brevis, insert threads transversely over the tendon sheath.

IV. Clinical Cases and Protocols

De Quervain's tenosynovitis

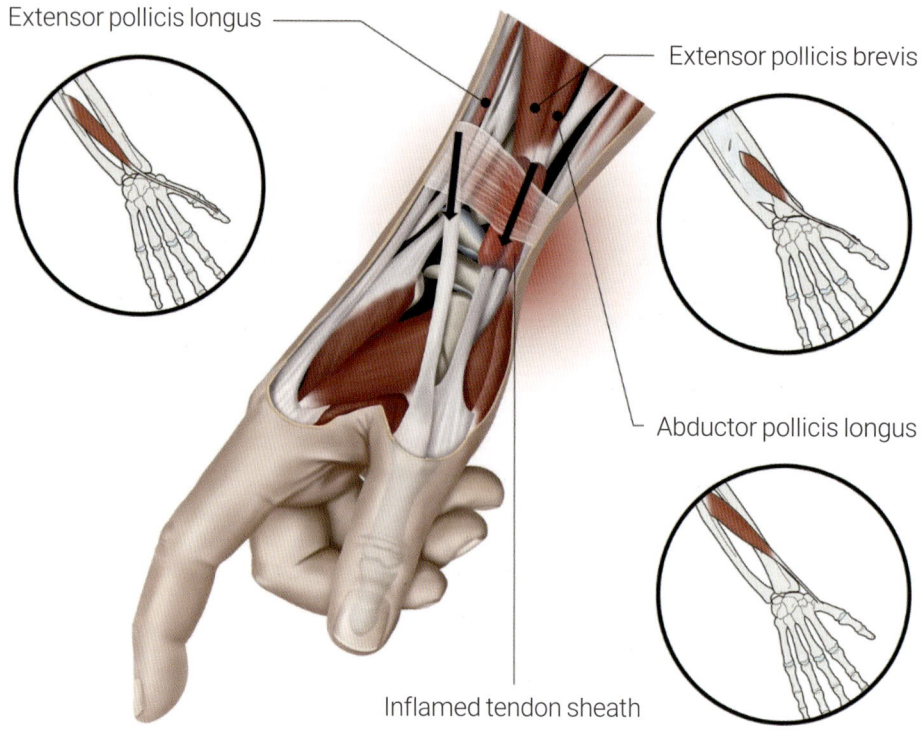

IV. Clinical Cases and Protocols

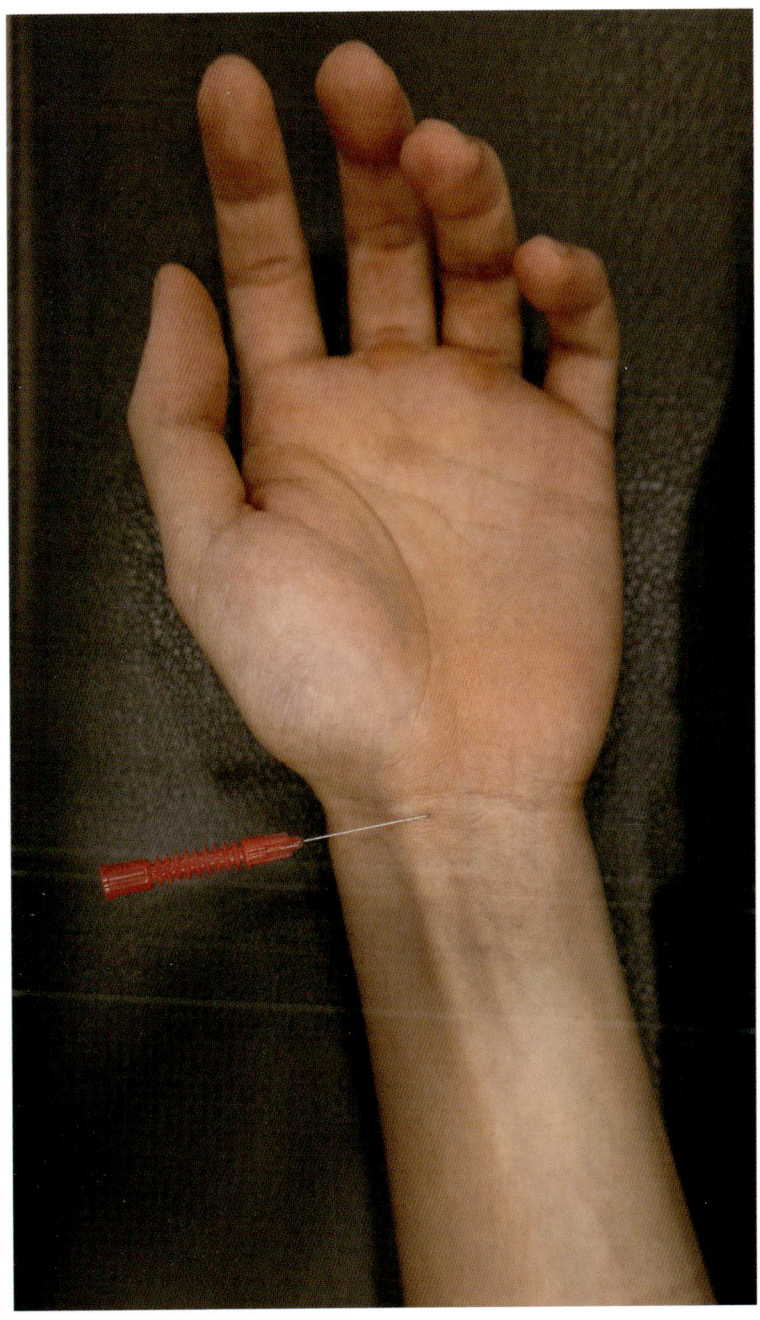

IV. Clinical Cases and Protocols

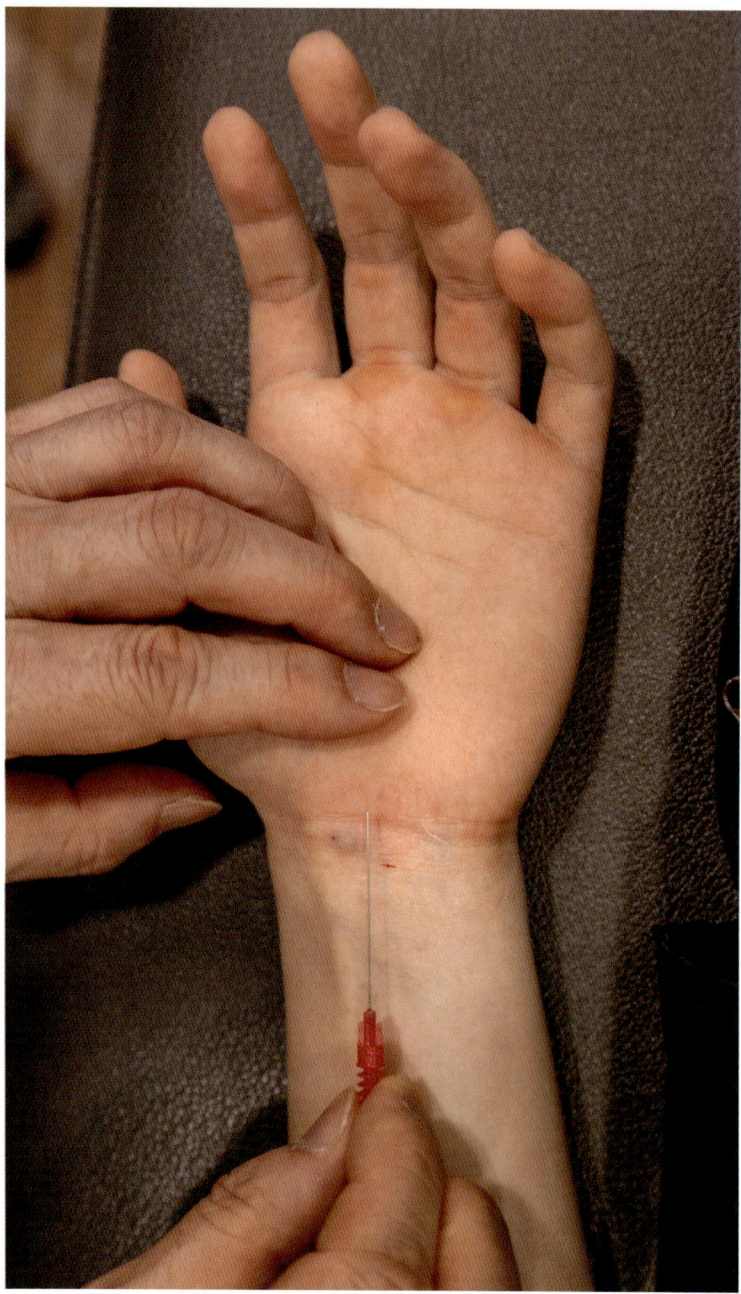

In cases of carpal tunnel syndrome, perform crosshatch thread embedding over the flexor retinaculum and administer pharmacopuncture concurrently.

IV. Clinical Cases and Protocols

Carpal Tunnel Syndrome

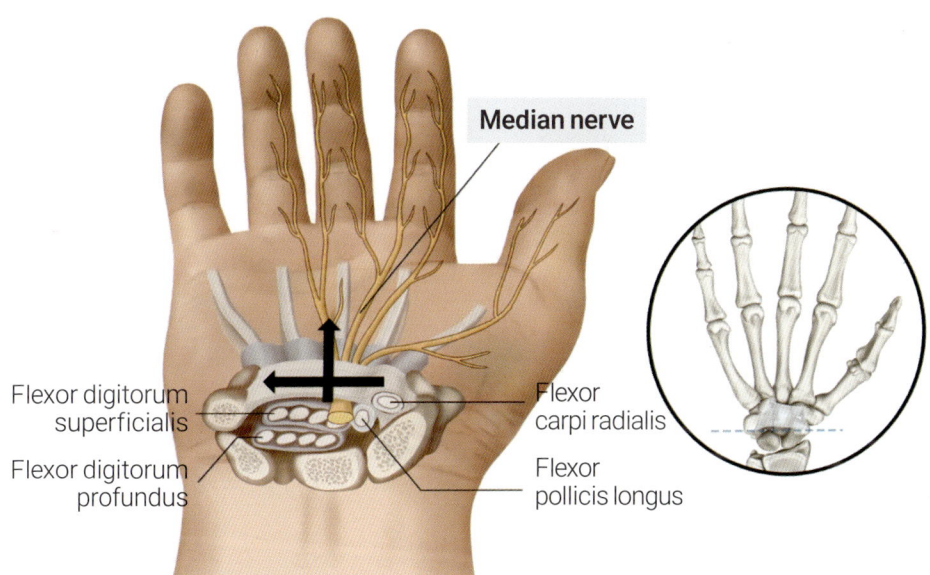

IV. Clinical Cases and Protocols

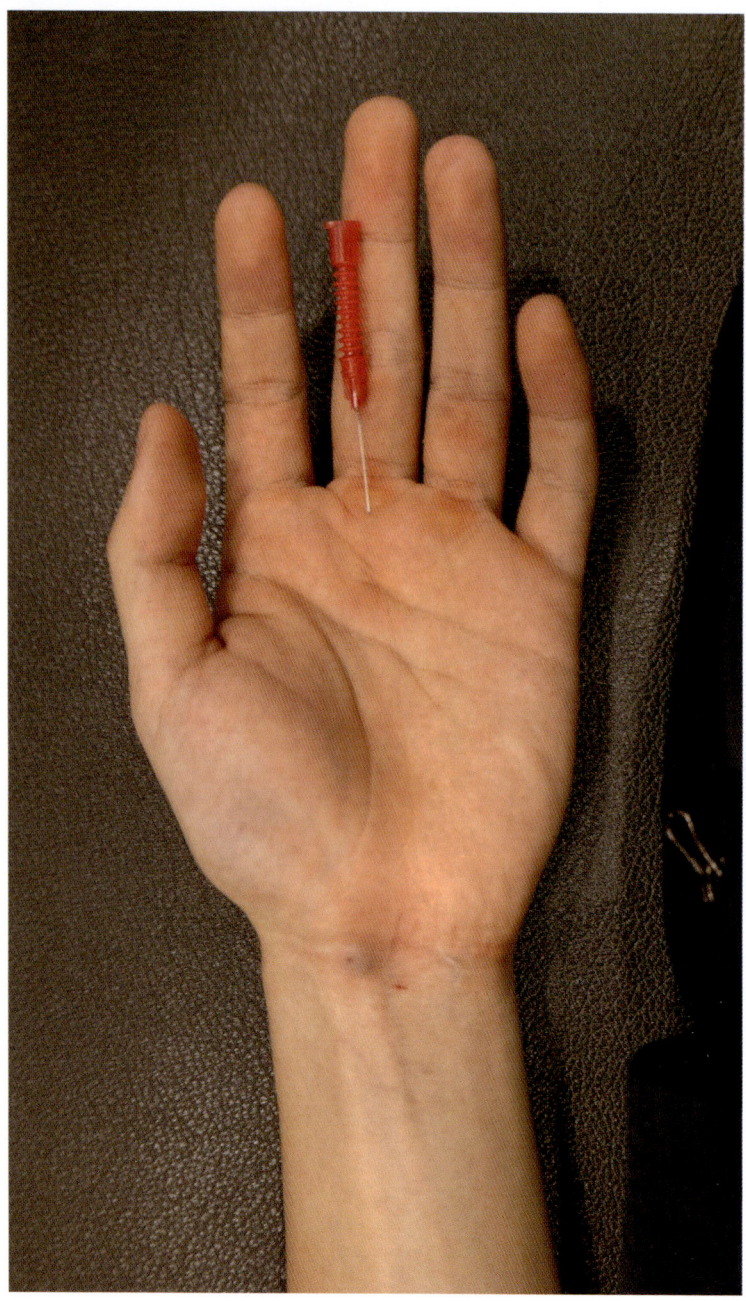

In cases of trigger finger, insert threads transversely over the tendon pulley region of the affected tendon.

IV. Clinical Cases and Protocols

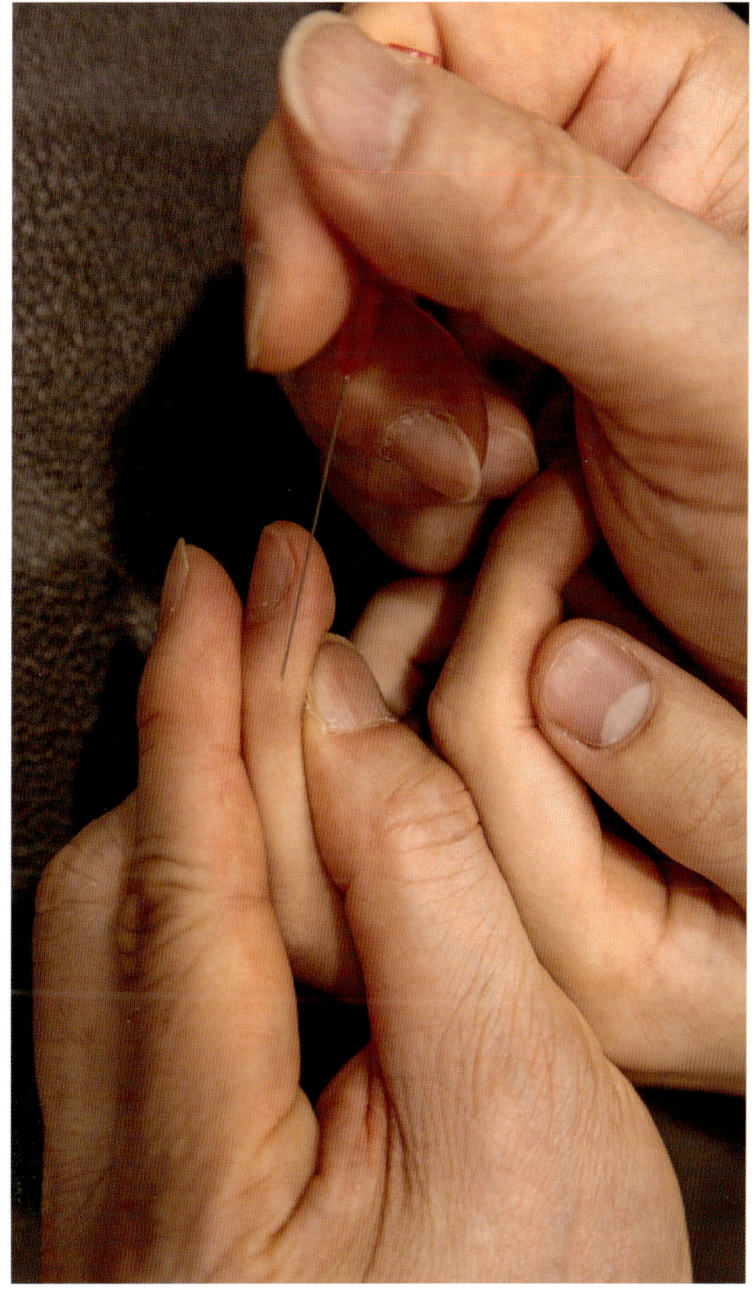

IV. Clinical Cases and Protocols

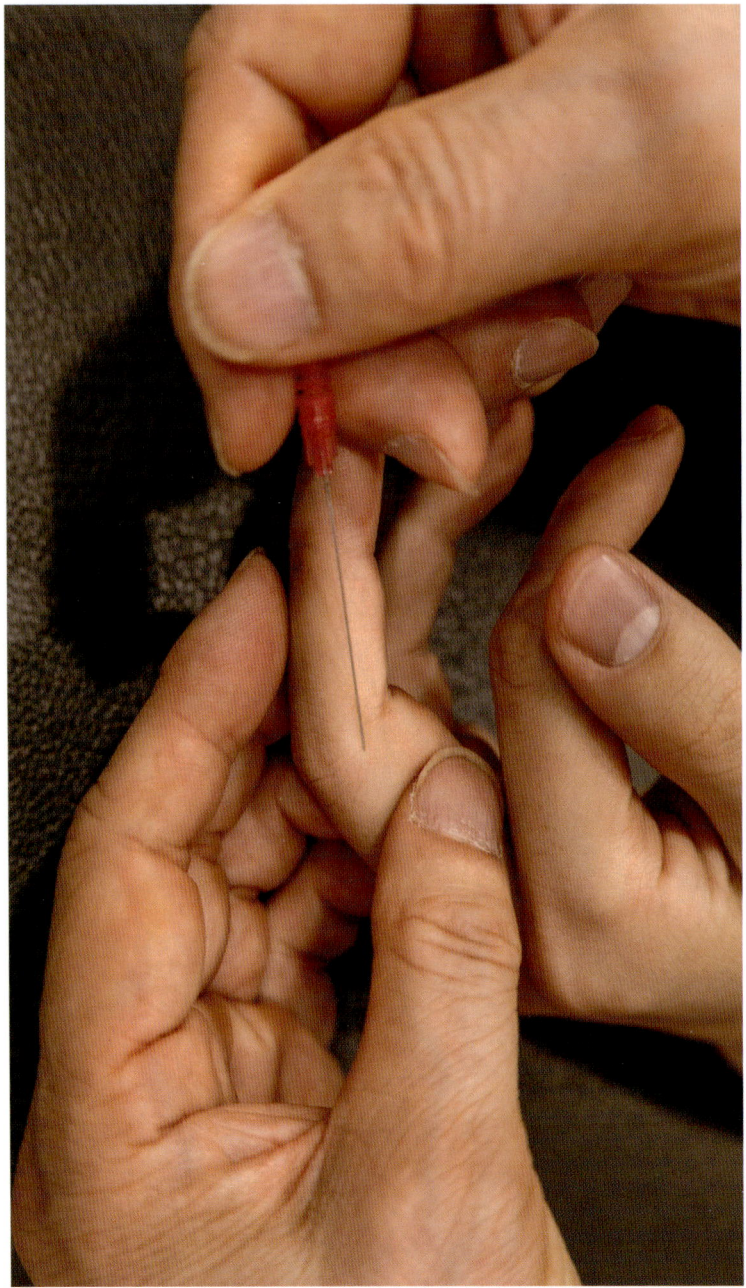

For finger joint arthritis or inflamed joints, perform thread embedding along the collateral ligaments of the affected joint.

V. Case Studies

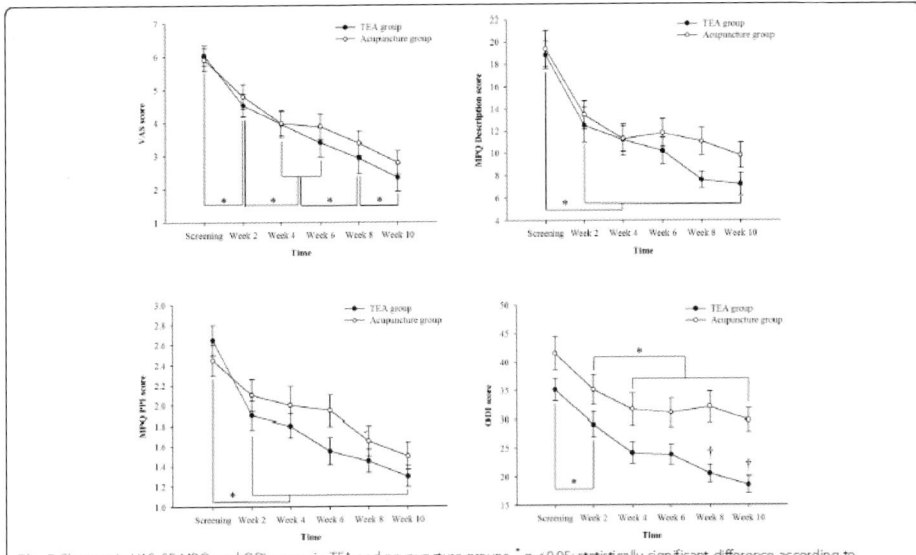

Fig. 5 Changes in VAS, SF-MPQ, and ODI scores in TEA and acupuncture groups. * $p < 0.05$: statistically significant difference according to repeated-measures analysis of variance (ANOVA) by contrast analysis with Bonferroni's correction on time. † $p < 0.05$: statistically significant difference according to repeated-measures analysis of variance (ANOVA) by contrast analysis with Bonferroni's correction on time and group interaction. *MPQ* short-form McGill Pain, *ODI* Oswestry Disability Index, *PPI* Present Pain Intensity scale, *TEA* thread-embedding acupuncture, *VAS* visual analog scale

According to the results of a randomized controlled pilot clinical trial conducted by Lee (2018) and colleagues, Thread Embedding Acupuncture may be both effective and safe for patients with chronic low back pain.

The key findings are as follows:
- Pain Reduction: Thread Embedding Acupuncture significantly reduced pain intensity in patients with chronic low back pain, as measured by the Visual Analog Scale (VAS).
- Functional Improvement: The therapy had a positive impact on functional disability, indicating an improved ability to perform daily activities that were previously limited by pain.
- Safety: The study demonstrated that Thread Embedding Acupuncture can be applied safely without serious adverse events. Most reported side effects were mild and temporary.

This study provides important preliminary evidence supporting the use of Thread Embedding Acupuncture as a relatively safe treatment that positively impacts both pain relief and functional improvement in patients with chronic low back pain.

VI. References

1. LEE KH, Lee DH, Kwon KR, et al. A Literary Study on Embedding Therapy. Journal of Pharmacopuncture. 2003;6:15-21.
2. Jung IH, Yun WH. The acupuncture for beauty and needle embedding. Seoul: Hansol. 2014.
3. Kwon K. The Analysis on the Present Condition of Thread Embedding Therapy Papers Published in Journal of Korean Medicine. Journal of Korean Medicine Ophthalmology & Otolaryngology & Dermatology. 2014;27:16-44.
4. Huo J, Zhao J, Yuan Y, et al. Research Status of the Effect Mechanism on Catgut-point Embedding Therapy. Chin Acupunct Moxib. 2017;37:1251-4.
5. Ha SH. Total Sling Medicine. 1st ed. Paju: Koonja Publishing Inc.; 2020:30-4.
6. Huang CY, Choong MY, Li TS. Treatment of Obesity by Catgut Embedding: An Evidence-Based Systematic Analysis. Acupunct Med. 2012;30(3):233-4.
7. Lee YJ. Mechanism of Chronic Pain and Interventional Neuro-Muscular Stimulation. Korean J Fam Med. 2006;27(5):341-51.
8. Song MY, Kim HJ. Recent Research Trends in Thread Embedding Therapy Applied to Obesity Treatment. J Korean Orient Med Obes. 2012;12(2):1-11.
9. Kim SH. Definition and Classification of Pain. Korean J Pain. 2008;1(1):1-7.
10. Lee YS, Jang MS, Kwon K. Analysis of Domestic and International Studies on Thread Embedding Therapy - Focusing on Clinical Studies -. J Prev Korean Med. 2016;20(1):93-113.
11. Yoon JH, Kim SS, Kim DI. Regenerative Medicine Using Physical Stimulation: Absorbable Threads. Seoul: MD World Publishing; 2017.
12. Jun P, Liu Y, Park JE, et al. Research Trends on the Thread Embedding Therapy of Low Back Pain in Traditional Chinese Medicine - Focusing on published articles in China. J Physiol & Pathol Korean Med. 2017;31(1):25-35.
13. Kang KW, Park JY, Kim JH, et al. Anti Wrinkle Effect of Needle-Embedding Therapy: a Case Series. J Korean Obstet Gynecol. 2018;31(1):147-54.
14. Nam EJ. Management and Approach to Patients with Chronic Pain. Korean J Med. 2007;73 Suppl 2:S794.
15. Yang J. A Study of Pain, Depression and Self-Efficacy According to the Classifications of Pain among Chronic Pain Patients. Korean J Adult Nurs. 2004;16(2):202-10.
16. Yu K, Kim J, Min S, et al. A Case Report of Patient with Recurrent Patellar Dislocation Treated by Korean Medicine Treatment in Combination with Intra-articular Bee Venom Injection and Needle Embedding Therapy. J Orient Rehabil Med. 2013;23(4):251-9.
17. Lee HJ, Choi BI, Jun S, et al. Efficacy and Safety of Thread-Embedding Acupuncture for Chronic Low Back Pain: A Randomized Controlled Pilot Trial. Trials. 2018;19(680):1-10.

VI. References

18. Kim JT, Choi SW, Han HJ, et al. A Literature Review and Recent Trends of Korean Medical Plastic Surgery and Thread Embedding Acupuncture. J Acupunct Moxib. 2009;26(6):131-42.
19. Han HJ, Kim MJ, Jang IS, et al. Three Cases of Hemiplegia after Stroke Treated by Thread Embedding Acupuncture on Scalp Acupoints. J Acupunct Moxib. 2013;30(5):313-23.
20. Min YG, Lim HG, Lee HJ, et al. Analysis of Recent Research Trends in Thread Embedding Acupuncture for Low Back Pain. J Acupunct Res. 2024;41(2):96-106.
21. Kim JH, Lee SM. Biodegradation Process of PCL Threads and Collagen Stimulation in Rat Models. J Aesthet Dermatol. 2022;15(3):45-52.
22. Yoon JH, Kim SS, Oh SM, Kim BC, Jung W. Tissue changes over time after polydioxanone thread insertion: An animal study with pigs. J Cosmet Dermatol. 2019;18(3):885-91.
23. Lee Y, Choi M. Foreign Body Reaction Patterns in Absorbable Thread Lift Procedures: Clinical Analysis of 500 Cases. Dermatol Surg. 2020;46(7):893-9.
24. Global Aesthetic Research Group. Multi-center Study on Thread Lift Complications : A 5-year Retrospective Analysis. Aesthet Plast Surg. 2023;47(1):78-85.
25. Yun YH, Kim TY, Lim TJ, et al. Narrative Review and Propose of Thread Embedding Acupuncture Procedure for Facial Wrinkles and Facial Laxity. J Korean Med Ophthalmol Otolaryngol Dermatol. 2015;28(1):112-25.
26. Frizziero A, Pellizzon G, Vittadini F, et al. Efficacy of Core Stability in Non-Specific Chronic Low Back Pain. J Funct Morphol Kinesiol. 2021;6(2):37.
27. Saini N, Tiwari S, Singh L. Evaluating the Impact of Cervical Stabilisation Exercises on Chronic Neck Pain: A Systematic Review. Musculoskeletal Care. 2025;23(2):e70091.
28. Standring S, ed. Gray's Anatomy: The Anatomical Basis of Clinical Practice. 41st ed. Philadelphia: Elsevier; 2016.
29. Moore KL, Dalley AF, Agur AM. Clinically Oriented Anatomy. 8th ed. Philadelphia: Wolters Kluwer; 2018.
30. Korean Medical Ophthalmology Otolaryngology & Dermatology Society. Analysis of the Therapeutic Mechanism of Thread Embedding Therapy in Korean Traditional Medicine Aesthetics. J Korean Med Ophthalmol Otolaryngol Dermatol. 2023;36(4):113-21.
31. Kang JI, Lee DH. Clinical Research Trends of Thread Embedding Acupuncture for Allergic Rhinitis. J Korean Med Ophthalmol Otolaryngol Dermatol. 2020;33(2):55-69.
32. Kim YJ, Jang GT, Lee SH. A Literature Review on Thread Embedding Therapy for Pediatric Enuresis: Focusing on Chinese Medicine Papers. J Korean Orient Pediatr. 2024;38(3):1-12.

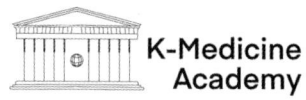

Hands-On Thread Embedding Therapy:
A Manual for Chronic Pain Treatment Through Structural Stabilization

First edition, first printing: September 10, 2025
First edition, first published: September 10, 2025

Writers: Byung-il Choi, Serin Lee, Seung Hwan Lee
Illustrator: Kyungmin Chu

Model: Junhyung Jung
Photographer: Sang Hee Cho
Materials provided by: Dongbang Medical Co., Ltd.
Planning: Heewon Lee, Joong-Han So

Publisher: Seung Hwan Lee
Editing & Design: Indiprint

Published by: K-Medicine Academy
Publication Registration Number: 2023-000165
Website: https://blog.naver.com/k-medicine-academy
Email: wooricare@naver.com

ISBN 979-11-986223-5-8(93510)

Copyright © 2025 by K-Medicine Academy
All rights reserved. No part of this publication may be reproduced without written permission from the publisher. The Publisher takes no responsibility for the use of the materials or methods described in this book nor for products thereof.